PATIENTS ARE PEOPLE

Patients Are People

A MEDICAL-SOCIAL APPROACH

TO PROLONGED ILLNESS

By Minna Field

THIRD EDITION

Columbia University Press
NEW YORK AND LONDON

Library of Congress Catalog Card Number: 67-31049
Printed in the United States of America

To THINKING AND FEELING PEOPLE

IN EVERY CENTURY

WHOSE FOCUS WAS THE VALUE OF HUMAN LIFE

AND THE NEED TO PROTECT AND CHERISH

EVERY ASPECT OF IT

FOREWORD

THE LENGTHENING SPAN OF LIFE, resulting from the great gifts of modern laboratory medicine, is of expanding significance as modern history unfolds to our eager gaze. Exercising pressure which derives its strength from the disproportion between somatic longevity and an adequate social response, it has been bringing physician and social worker together to the end that longer life may be achieved more happily and made worthy of the common effort. In this endeavor we find youth serving age, and so healing a breach which has brought much unhappiness to both by its persistence through the generations. This reconciliation is one of the major by-products of the new specialty of social medicine.

For one thing, age is a cumulative phenomenon, medically speaking. Very few enter the late period who have not had their lives prolonged by the health and medical benefactions which are now part of our heritage—a boon which has been conferred on them by the grace of their fellow men, in war and in peace. Others have pulled themselves up by their own bootstraps, unaided, and still others become old in spite of lingering illness. Many people take a long and heartbreaking time to die as prolonged illness clings to them during the less resistant age periods. Constitutional factors are more decisive in the earlier age periods since they serve to restrain or modify the invading illness. There is, therefore, a strong affinity between age and disease which men naturally fear.

The gradual subtraction of the joys of life with the addition of years alters the delicate balance to which most people have been accustomed. As the rights, privileges, and immunities of youth fade with the passage of time, this biological transition is accompanied either by a spirit of resignation or of resistance, as the case may be. When illness is superimposed on an organism handicapped by age, we have a social problem of the first magnitude. Prolonged illness, sad enough in youth, is much more sad if only because it is much more extensive and of longer duration when it is entangled with age. Socially and medically—and how can the two be considered apart from each other?—prolonged illness in the later years, when people should be privileged to look back in comfort on a life well spent, is the ultimate curse. Than this there is no greater challenge to our planning efforts.

It is in the midst of such a human problem that the author of this volume has been spending her professional life. We would do well to listen carefully to her analysis of her findings and give heed to her contribution to the sum total of the effort that is our common duty. In spite of the pretensions of philanthropy, we are still confronted with the restraints of inertia in the midst of the glowing embers which are being blown in all directions from the conflagration of disease. Unreasonable fear of the loss of individual or organizational identity has been having a deadly effect on those who are afflicted with prolonged illness. In the competitive arena where rewards for such effort are distributed as prizes, men seem to be playing a game with the methods which have brought them success elsewhere. It is to the nobler side of the philanthropic nature—to its pristine goodness—that the author appeals in these pages. And she leaves no doubt in our minds that there is much yet to be done to make longer life worth the effort to acquire it.

E. M. Bluestone, m.d.

FOREWORD TO THE
SECOND EDITION

No better statement of the aims of rehabilitation has been made than the words of the philosopher Paulsen when he said, "The object of all help is to make help superfluous." For the chronically ill and disabled, this is more than a polite statement; it is an article of faith.

Because rehabilitation deals with the whole person, it has a definite place in any discussion of the concept that "patients are people." People are not only sick persons, amputees, or paraplegics, they are doctors, engineers, teachers, artisans, and poets. They are graduates of high school; they live in metropolitan communities or country suburbs; they are single; they are married; they have children as well as hopes, aims, and aspirations for the future. These and thousands of others hunger not only for relief from long-term illness, but, more important, for independence and personal dignity.

Today, we know that this independence can be achieved, not only because of the development of new techniques, but primarily because of the vast potentials in the disabled. These human resources can now be tapped and developed into constructive channels. Unfortunately, too much emphasis has been placed upon a job or earning capacity as the specific goal of rehabilitation. While a substantial number of the chronically ill and disabled can be restored to gainful employment, the greatest satisfaction comes from teaching the individual to become personally independent. In our preoccupation with making the handicapped person again employable, we have overlooked the tremendous social and psychological and even economic benefits that come from self-help activities.

All these facts have been brought forward by the author in a careful and thoughtful way. She has condensed in a meaningful manner the essential facts and principles which have brought the impact of rehabilitation to its present importance in the field of health and social welfare.

HENRY H. KESSLER, M.D.

Cʜʀᴏɴɪᴄ ɪʟʟɴᴇss ʀᴇᴍᴀɪɴᴇᴅ for a long period an unexplored territory, and those who attempted to explore it had to overcome both basic ignorance of its nature as well as lack of skills to deal with the problems it presented. A more subtle obstruction to action, however, was the refusal—intentional or unintentional—by society to recognize the very existence of a problem and consequently of the need to do anything about it. The cliché that "what we don't know doesn't concern us" served as justification for inaction and contentment with the *status quo*. The medical profession contributed to the neglect of this group of sick people by its continued emphasis on the needs of the acutely ill.

This neglect persisted until the civilized world progressed beyond the point where an entire group could be ignored and treated negatively, if at all. At first the provisions for the care of the chronically ill were determined primarily by society's emotional reaction to a group of people whom they saw as old, crippled, dependent, incurable, and indigent. In its desire to remove itself from the emotional impact this created, society made provision for "these people" to be put in "special" facilities where presumably they could receive "special" care.

The persistent concern of interested individuals began to be felt, although slowly. At first, the approach to the problem and the programs to deal with it were segmented on the basis of diagnostic categories, age levels, and socioeconomic conditions. It was only as knowledge accumulated and a better understanding of chronic illness was developed that it became recognized that the multifaceted problems which these patients presented required an integrated, multidiscipline approach. At the same time, it became apparent that the understanding of the past as it affected the presenting disability was essential to insure effective treatment. This understanding led to the recognition that a continuum of care must be developed from acute illness through all phases of extended care, including rehabilitation as a means of treatment of the end result of chronic disability. In this process, it was felt, not only the patient himself, but the family, the community, and the professional personnel required skilled help.

There still remain largely uncharted regions of research and education waiting for discovery by the investigator and academician to become mutually involved as explorers with the clinician.

When knowledge and wisdom are developed, progress will be immobilized without those who have the capacity to transmit not only the revelations of history and current understanding, but also the philosophic stimulus to guarantee continued generations of explorers. The author has the curiosity to learn, the capacity to integrate the composite picture, the drive to persist, and most important of all—the generosity to share by teaching with those who become her heirs.

JAMES C. HART, M.D.

ACKNOWLEDGMENTS

I WISH TO EXPRESS my deep appreciation to Dr. E. M. Bluestone for his careful editing of the first draft of the book. In his capacity as Director of Montefiore Hospital, Dr. Bluestone has guided the hospital for over twenty years. Without the inspiration he provided, the philosophy embodied in this book could not have been formulated.

My thanks go, also, to Dr. Henry H. Kessler for his Foreword to the second edition. I am grateful for this expression of Dr. Kessler's viewpoint, based, as it is, on many years of working with handicapped people.

To Ethel H. Wise, chairman of the Social Service Committee, go my thanks for her unfailing support in making the philosophy of total medical care a living reality by facilitating the integration of the social services with medical care, thus assuring for the patient the benefit of a thoughtful consideration of all problems confronting him.

Professor Gordon Hamilton, of the New York School of Social Work of Columbia University, has my heartfelt appreciation for the thoughtful reading of the manuscript and for the many valuable suggestions which helped to accentuate and clarify the points made and improved immeasurably the organization of the material.

Special thanks are due to my colleagues on the staff of the Social Service Department of Montefiore Hospital, whose daily performance in the carrying out of their duties is a living embodiment of the philosophy enunciated in this book and who, through case material and discussion, helped to crystallize my thinking. Special mention needs to be made of Mrs. Bess S. Dana and Mrs. Juliette C. Lipeles, who had an active part in the early formulation of the plans and in drawing up the original text of what is now the first chapter. And to my husband, Jacob, whose unfailing understanding and warm support eased many moments of frustration and discouragement, goes my sincere appreciation.

MINNA FIELD

ACKNOWLEDGMENTS

TO THE THIRD EDITION

I AM INDEBTED TO Dr. James C. Hart, Director of the Restoration Center of the Veterans Administration Hospital in East Orange, New Jersey, for his willingness to share with me his philosophy of total restoration of the patient and for his careful reading of the portion of this edition describing the function of the Restoration Center.

Miss Barbara G. Schutt, R.N., editor of the *American Journal of Nursing*, was particularly helpful in contributing to my understanding of the present-day thinking regarding the educational requirement for nurses.

My thanks to Dr. Martin Cherkasky, Director of Montefiore Hospital of New York, and his staff for helping me get acquainted with the latest developments in medical care at the hospital.

CONTENTS

PATIENTS ARE PEOPLE

I

INTRODUCTORY
STATEMENT

It is generally recognized that the present-day practice of total medical care is predicated on the appreciation of the interrelationship of social, emotional, and pathological forces in the care of the sick. This book endeavors to portray the integration of this understanding into actual practice. The philosophy it propounds is, in a sense, as old as the Biblical injunction that "the care of the sick is a sacred task" and as new as the photographic reproductions of the effects of emotion on bodily functions.

Since the aim of this book is to be more logical than chronological, I have purposely refrained from a factual discussion of historical developments in social work in general, and medical social work in particular. There are many books devoted to this subject. My discussion centers rather on the evolution of a concept of integration of medical and social care of the sick which was influenced more deeply by increased understanding of human behavior and by broad social changes than by any single historical fact. In line with this aim, my concern is not always with who did what, when, and why, but how much what was done has affected and changed our manner of thinking about illness and the sick person.

The case material presented and the concepts formulated are based on the experiences of the author gained in a large voluntary general hospital devoted to the care and treatment of patients with prolonged illness. While the emphasis, conditioned as it is by the author's experience and interest, is primarily on prolonged illness, the principles formulated are applicable to the treatment of sick people everywhere regardless of the diagnosis or the duration of the illness.

EVOLUTION OF A CONCEPT

Montefiore Hospital in New York City was for many years the only voluntary general hospital in the United States devoted exclusively to the scientific study and treatment of prolonged illness (exclusive of mental conditions). Founded in 1884 as a "home for chronic invalids," the institution developed in response to changing medical and social philosophies. Now, a general voluntary hospital, it stands, as it did in the past, in the forefront of progressive thinking and planning for medical-social care of patients. In its prime scientific facilities, Montefiore Hospital is the living proof that the distinction between "acute" and "chronic" illnesses and the different treatment accorded them in the past are no longer valid.

The advanced thinking which characterized Montefiore's approach to the needs of the patient and the type of care he required is evident throughout the years of its existence. From the very beginning the hospital, influenced by the faith and inspiration of a few community leaders not content merely to provide an "asylum for the needy sick," emphasized "the treatment of disease as opposed to a shelter for the doomed." [1] The first medical report issued a year after the founding of the institution illustrates this attitude. The report stated that "49 persons had been treated, of whom 13 were discharged, 3 as cured, 4 as improved." [2] This simple statement assumes a new significance when one considers that it was written in an age which knew nothing of x-rays, radium, or cobalt and which was inclined to view the "chron-

---

[1] Bracker, p. 5.   [2] *Ibid.*

ics" as hopeless and not expected to respond to medical treatment.

This different attitude, which refused to succumb to the prevalent hopelessness, made itself felt in yet another direction. Montefiore Hospital, beginning as a small institution, early identified itself not only with the cases of the relatively few patients it could serve within its walls, but also with the larger problem of prolonged illness as it affected others beyond the hospital's intramural care. Recognizing the paucity of available knowledge so far as prolonged illness was concerned, the hospital encouraged scientific research as part of its program almost from the very beginning. In the course of the years that have passed since its establishment, the scientists associated with the institution distinguished themselves as pioneers in the development of many new methods of treatment of prolonged illness in all its phases. Such emphasis on the scientific aspects of care when applied to prolonged illness at that particular point in the development of medical care in general could only spring from a fundamental respect for the value of the individual human being, since the patients under the care of Montefiore Hospital represented that part of the sick population whom society as a whole had been inclined to relegate to a human scrap heap at a distance.

It is not surprising that in such an environment, with its emphasis on the intrinsic worth of the patient as a person, interest was centered not merely on the disease process, but on the patient as a person and on his social background as well. As early as 1885 the Ladies Auxiliary Society was formed and devoted itself to the performance of personal services to the patients in the hospital. What is even more significant, the members visited each new applicant for admission in order to make "intelligent and sympathetic decisions" regarding his suitability. The emphasis on the need to make "intelligent" decisions indicates a recognition of the value of knowing as much as possible about the patient. Even more important is the use of the word "sympathetic," for it implies an understanding of the meaning the patient's social situation may have for him and of the need to take it into consideration. The philosophy expressed by this concern with "intelligent and sympathetic decisions" is as valid today as it was in 1885, and a tribute to these people of good will whose activities made an important contribution to the concepts which form the basis of modern professional thinking and practice along more orderly, systematic lines.

As was to be expected in a hospital whose primary emphasis was on the patient's total needs, a social service department was established early. From its inception it became an integral part of the services the hospital stood ready to provide. As we look back to the nineteenth century we find that these social workers were, in a sense, ahead of their times. In that particular period in history, the profession of social work in general, following the lead of the medical profession, concentrated on providing services to the acutely ill whose prognosis was hopeful. By contrast to the prevailing attitude, the social workers attached to this particular hospital, devoted to the care of the least hopeful group among the sick, did not allow the prognosis for the patient with whom they worked to prejudice them against seeing the person behind the illness or to influence their efforts on his behalf. Throughout, their activities indicated a guiding philosophy which emphasized the intrinsic worth and dignity of the human being. Despite this broader vision, they were nevertheless circumscribed in rendering the necessary help since the skill they possessed was determined by the level of development in the field of social work as a whole. Their techniques were sharpened only as social work grew and unfolded professionally.

This was the setting and the beginning of an institution

which has evolved over the years a program of total integration of medical-social care of its patients. The implications of such an integrated approach will be discussed in detail in the pages that follow.

2

EVOLUTION OF
A CONCEPT

CHRONIC, long-term, or, better still, "prolonged" illness has been receiving increased attention in recent years as the major medical-social problem of our time. In an era characterized by dramatic victories over disease in general, the rising incidence of prolonged illness presents a challenge to everyone concerned with the provision of adequate care for the sick. Paradoxically enough, the very advances made by medical science left us with the problem of a large residue of prolonged illness. The curtailment of infant mortality, the reduction in the fatal outcome of many of the infectious diseases, the practical elimination of epidemics, all these mean that more people live longer. Though children and young adults are not immune from the ravages of prolonged illness, the number so afflicted is higher in the older age group, for the longer people live, the greater the likelihood of their developing one of the slow-moving, degenerative, or malignant illnesses which frequently accompany the process of aging and the longer the period that these illnesses will persist. The challenge that confronts us now is how to provide adequate care for a large number of patients over a prolonged period of time and how to succeed where we have hitherto failed, both in prevention and treatment.

THE NATURE OF PROLONGED ILLNESS

What is prolonged illness? While it escapes exact medical definition, it is perhaps most accurately described by Dr.

E. M. Bluestone, who speaks of it in this way: "Prolonged illness should be viewed for all practical purposes as an extension of acute disease over a longer period of time." This definition captures a philosophy that is broader than the time element alone and embraces the concept of treatability of the illness, no matter what its phase and regardless of its stubbornness. In the light of such a concept, the establishment of a diagnosis of prolonged illness no longer carries with it the primary implication of medical hopelessness, imminent death, or lifelong invalidism, as the term "chronic" did in the past. On the contrary, as in any other illness, the diagnosis is seen as but the first step toward treatment. The emphasis is no longer on whether or not to treat the patient in the face of a prognosis of incurability, but on how best to treat him with every facility at our disposal. Prolonged illness is not a separate entity. The general term "prolonged illness" includes many illnesses with different etiologies, different symptomatologies, different effects on each patient—no two patients being exactly alike—and requiring different treatment procedures.

Neither is prolonged illness a universally hopeless, static condition. Its very nature implies a continuity of the disease, calling for a continuity in treatment. Changes in the patient's condition often occur. These changes are related to the four phases of the disease: the acute phase, in which active medical care within a hospital is imperative; the convalescent stage in which the patient prepares for a return to normal or near normal health; the chronic stage in which the patient can function in his normal environment, provided he recognizes his limitations and receives continued medical and nursing supervision; and the custodial stage, in which the patient requires care with a minimum of medical attention. These steps do not necessarily follow one another in this order in the course of any one illness. The patient in the chronic stage of his illness may experience an acute exacerbation of symptoms, necessitating rehospitalization and active medical intervention. The condition of the custodial patient may fluctuate to the degree that either he is able to take on more activity or he requires intensive medical treatment. At any one of the stages concurrent illnesses may develop and reqiure attention. Each phase of the illness carries with it special implications, presents special problems, and calls for special ways of meeting them. Because prolonged illness is viewed as a continuous and changing biological process with serious social implications, showing periods of remission, recovery, and acute exacerbation, each stage of the illness requires a different kind of care. The type of care is determined by the patient's physical condition, the degree of activity he is able to assume, and the amount and kind of help which must be supplied by others. Institutional care is only part of the answer during urgent phases of illness. An over-all institution for patients with prolonged illness is out of keeping with our present-day understanding of it.

The social implications of prolonged illness cannot be separated from their medical implications, and the problems which they jointly present seriously affect the patient, his family, the professional groups concerned with his care, and the community of which they are all a part.

CHANGES IN THE CONCEPT OF
MEDICAL CARE

This broadened concept of prolonged illness as both a medical and a social problem is a development of recent years and reflects the general tendency of modern medicine to consider the influence of social (including psychological) forces as contributory to pathological phenomena.

As we look back, we see the advances in the care of patients with prolonged illness subtly reflected in the changing nomenclature. Not so long ago, patients suffering from incapacitating illnesses over long periods of time were referred to as "custodial" and "incurable." Little was known about their ailments, what caused them or how to treat them. As a result, the family doctor, handicapped by limited medical knowledge in the care of the long-term sick, could do little for the patient except to administer psychological stimulants from time to time. Family members, unable to give the ill person even the most elementary physical care that his condition so frequently required, demanded that some provision be made outside the home. In this demand, the families expressed not only their difficulty in meeting the physical burden imposed by the illness, but even more their inability to carry the emotional burden it imposed and the feeling of helplessness evoked by the presence of the constantly sick person. As a result, the community tended to segregate the "incurables," whenever possible, in institutions away from the general hospitals and available medical facilities, such as they were, while the medical practitioners concentrated on treating those patients whom they knew how to help. In contrast, however, to the neglect which was associated with the medieval segregation of the hopelessly ill, we had, even in the era of the "incurables," a beginning awareness of the patient as a person, some appreciation of what the illness meant to him, and an awakening sense of responsibility for making the "incurable" as comfortable as possible through sedation, routine nursing care, diet, more cheerful surroundings, and a more hopeful atmosphere.

This changed emphasis in the management of the "incurables" was in line with the trend of the times. This was the era of benevolence. Ladies bountiful dispensed their baskets of goodies to the good, and frowned upon the nonconformists by withholding their gifts. History reflects, in every area, the same tendency to grant to the giver the prerogative of judging the worthiness of the receiver. Medicine, too, advanced through the concept of the "worthy" patient. Sometimes the patient was considered "worthy" because of the interesting aspects of the clinical picture he presented. At other times, a particular patient aroused the doctor's sympathy because of the extreme suffering he was undergoing. Again, a patient might be singled out because he had capitulated to his illness, suffered silently, expected little from others, and rewarded the medical personnel by being "good," uncomplaining and overtly grateful for whatever little was being done for him. While we today, concerned with the preservation of the rights of the individual and of human dignity, may question such an attitude, we must recognize that it served as a foundation for the advances that have since ensued. The combination of the right man of medical science at the right time for the right illness which satisfied his special interest came much later and by a very hard historic path.

Even though patients might have been singled out for attention because of their "worthiness," clinically or financially, the all-important fact remains that a beginning toward treatment was made. Because of their personal feelings of interest, sympathy, and concern for a particular patient in the "incurable" group, but more often because they were attracted to a problem with which they felt they could help, doctors began to employ methods of treatment which had proved their efficacy in the care of acutely ill patients. It was hoped that even if such treatment could not cure, it would at least alleviate the pain and discomfort of a so-called "incurable" patient. Sometimes the methods were successful. Then, even as today, the smallest particle of success served to stimulate the doctor's professional interest and to inspire him to new efforts on behalf of those who came to him for help. As these special, personalized efforts and increased attention brought results in some cases, the sense of achievement attained by the doctor, coupled with the capturing of his scientific interest, proved a sufficient stimulus to enlarge the scope of his endeavors to include, not only the patients whom he liked personally and, therefore, felt deserved care, but all others who might profit from his services.

There are no dramatic or specific examples of this change in attitude. A single doctor, observing the response of a single patient to the plus factor of treatment, in addition to custodial care, might engage the interest of another doctor in his activities. Step by step, as discoveries and methods of treatment of illness in general increased, an attempt was made to test their effectiveness on the permanently afflicted. With the stimulation which comes with success, and inspired by new discoveries and the expansion of actual medical knowledge, interest grew into the kind of conviction that eventually brought about the separation of the curables from the "chronic and custodial." The actual amount of medical attention remained minimal, and the facilities for care were still removed from centers of medical research and treatment. Nevertheless, the first step in the direction of scientific recognition of the treatability of the so-called "incurable" had been taken.

The time was ripe for such a step. The advent of the twentieth century brought with it far-reaching changes in the mode of living and, consequently, changes in the practice of medicine. In truth, the developments in medicine cannot be separated from the related development of the society in which it is practiced, for medicine, as one of the biological sciences, is a part of life. Wars, famines, and industrial revolutions not only bring in their wake disease, discomfort, unhappiness, and death, but, as we know from past experience, at the same time give impetus to new discoveries in methods of treatment.

The changes in the physical and social atmosphere of the new century brought with them profound changes in the concept of what constitutes an adequate program of medical care. The earlier philosophy of the survival of the fittest was replaced by a concern for the rights of the individual and the acceptance of responsibility for his welfare, no matter what his physical or intellectual endowments. Worthiness was no longer the only criterion for extending help when needed, for it was out of keeping with the philosophy of a democratic society to neglect even its least productive members. The medical profession, responding to this awakened social consciousness, moved toward a more active medical program for the care of the sick in general, and the patient with prolonged illness in particular.

We witness the development of the specialized hospital for the care of the chronically ill as part of this growing concern. The fate of the forgotten "chronic" patient had become a stench in the nostrils of society which could no longer be tolerated. The hospital for "chronic diseases" is a logical outgrowth of its historical antecedents. At first it retained many of the features of the custodial institution from which it evolved. Gradually it brought to the segregation of the past the latter-day concern with the patient as a person, and the adaptation of modern scientific methods to his care. Even when these scientific methods were applied, however, they were not only the last to be added, but also the least to be emphasized. It is only within our generation that the emphasis has shifted from "chronic" to "hospital" in the joint title, resulting eventually in the complete abandonment of the word "chronic" and its replacement by the designation "general."

At the same time, changes of far-reaching importance were occurring in the physical setting in which the medical man practiced his art, influencing profoundly the over-all trends in medical care. Practicing in the small, rural community, the old horse-and-buggy doctor knew his patients intimately, as well as the community in which they lived. An integral part of the community himself, he understood their family problems, their concerns about money, their fears about themselves. Practicing in an era of common sense, unaided by instruments of precision, he tended to dispense homilies instead of hormones and was often looked to as a family counselor as well as the family physician.

The development of the far-flung urban community created a physical separation of doctor from patient with resulting estrangement and less intimate knowledge of the patient's total life situation. This physical estrangement, coupled with the rapid expansion of medical knowledge, which inevitably led to an equally rapid growth of specialization, confined many doctors to the treatment of a specific area of the body. Such specialization with its concentration on the sick organ served to obscure the fundamental concept of the patient as a total human being. As a result, we find that the doctor nowadays is likely to know a great deal more about the pathology of his patients than did his predecessors, but is less apt to know what his patient is really like as a person, who his family is, what his children are like, where he works, what he gets from his job, how he lives, and what he lives for.

We hear a great deal these days about psychosomatic medicine and the influence of emotions on the patient's physical condition. And yet the concept of the patient as a whole person is, in reality, not new. It was recognized long ago that one cannot separate the sick organ from the person to whom the organ belongs, as is attested by the age-old adage that "the part can never be well unless the whole is well." Nor is the concept of interrelation between physical and emotional states new. *Mens sana in corpore sano* is as old as, if not older than, the Roman Empire. Paradoxically enough, it is the medical practitioner, the one man most intimately concerned with the health of the patient, who, while learning more and more about the illness he is treating, has come to know less and less about the person who has the illness.

CHANGES IN THE CONCEPT OF
SOCIAL SERVICE

Fortunately, this appears to have been but a transient period in the development of the science of medicine. Present-day

thinking recognizes that sound, comprehensive medical treatment presupposes not only a knowledge of the physical
pathology, but also of the social factors, their effect upon the
patient, his illness, and his response to medical care. The old
dictum that "it is as important to know what kind of patient
has the disease as what kind of disease the patient has" has
been revitalized and has taken on new significance. An
awakened social conscience, the growth of democratic ideals,
the increase in medical knowledge, and the development of a
better understanding of interrelation between the psyche and
the soma, all have contributed to an appreciation of the need
for a better utilization of such a comprehensive approach.

The modern medical practitioner, confronted by his inability to assimilate the ever expanding accumulation of new
and complex medical knowledge and techniques, recognizes
his need for help from specialists in the various fields to
enrich his understanding of the patient's medical pathology.
In the same way, the complexity of modern living makes it
impossible for him to be knowledgeable in all the factors
which impinge upon the lives and health of his patients, or to
handle, as he so often did in the past, the numerous problems
which prolonged illness creates for him. Confronted with
these problems he has learned to look for help in understanding the social pathology of the patient, its possible bearing upon the medical picture, and the way in which the
strengths inherent in the social situation can be counted
upon to facilitate the fight against illness.

The profession of medical social work thus evolved as a
direct response to this desire on the part of the doctor to
know more about the social, economic, and family problems
his patients face, as well as his need to get help with these
problems so as to make it possible for the patient to maintain
the benefits he derives from medical treatment.

As we look back upon the development of social work, we
see that the social worker, like the doctor, tended in the

beginning to concentrate on patients with an acute illness whose recovery was most likely. At first, her attitude toward patients with prolonged illness, influenced by the medical profession, to which she looked for leadership, was one of futility. What could she do when the doctors could do so little? Wasn't she perfectly justified, she reasoned, in conserving her efforts, and the small philanthropic funds available to her, for the most hopeful cases?

When social work was first introduced into the general scheme of hospital organization, the social worker was a volunteer with interest in the "underprivileged." Her contribution was, primarily, in rendering friendly services to make the patient's stay in the hospital more endurable, to bring him some measure of cheer and comfort. When the professional social worker first replaced the volunteer, the duties were somewhat expanded, though the emphasis remained essentially the same. The worker continued to be primarily concerned with maintaining a friendly contact, with providing simple, concrete services. She helped to carry out the medical recommendations by supplying dentures and eyeglasses to those who could not afford to buy these things. She looked for a job for the patient whose illness had forced him to give up his usual work and who was not functionally able to resume his former activity. She was an expert in locating a convalescent home for the patient who needed a few weeks of rest following hospitalization.

As she performed these services, the social worker had an opportunity to observe that different patients reacted differently, not only to the medical treatment provided by the hospital but also to the services she was offering. Inspired by her discoveries of the highly individualized reactions, she began to realize that the things she was learning about people were being talked about and written about by the growing profession of psychiatry. She found in the psychiatric lectures and writings much that she could apply helpfully to her own job, so that her role began to take on new significance and to make increasing demands for greater knowledge and skill on her part.

Later, we see her beginning to question why one patient consistently broke his glasses, why another always had an excuse for not wearing the dentures secured for him, why a third left the convalescent home before the two weeks were over. The psychiatric lectures she attended and the books she read helped her to see that what she had in the past considered as unreasonable, perverse, or uncooperative behavior could be better understood if seen as symptomatic of some deeper, underlying problem. It then became apparent that the broken glasses, the troublesome dentures, the abandoned convalescent home, were neither mere accidents nor indications of a deliberate intent on the part of the patient to be contrary. Rather, they were evidence of some inner or outer difficulty the patient had in carrying out the medical recommendation. The social worker began to see her role as not merely supplying the patient with what was medically recommended for him, but as helping him overcome the underlying difficulties, and so making it possible for him to use constructively the services she was able to provide. Despite this growing understanding, the social worker's usefulness continued for some time to be limited and mainly confined to the patient whose prospect for recovery was most hopeful.

Unfortunately, or fortunately, the realities of everyday living disrupted the complacency of her rationalization. The strict lines of demarcation between "acute" and "chronic" that were built up around her were being abolished by sheer force of circumstances. The patient with an acute episode of his chronic condition frequently found his way into a general hospital for acute illnesses. Long after his acute medical need had been successfully overcome, he continued to occupy an urgently needed bed because his residual handicap made it impossible for him to be cared for at home. Because of her knowledge of community resources, it was natural that the social worker should be called upon to help with the post-hospital care of these patients, and thus free beds for the more acutely ill. The more closely she worked with patients suffering from prolonged illness, the more aware she became that these patients differed one from another as much as they, as a group, differed from the acutely ill patients. It became increasingly apparent that the differences in the reactions she observed had their roots in individual personalities rather than in disease groups. Just as the doctors had learned that the methods of treatment which brought alleviation and cure to the patient with acute illness could often be successfully applied to patients with prolonged illness, so did the social worker discover that her understanding and skill, developed in serving acutely ill patients, were equally applicable to the problems presented by patients with prolonged illness. As patients began to respond to therapy, and in line with the increase in medical optimism, the social worker too was inspired to help the patient achieve a social gain commensurate with his physical progress. The manifold social, emotional, and economic problems created by the residual effects of prolonged illness, for which medical science could do little, offered the greatest challenge to her professional skills.

The introduction of the professional social worker into the medical team caring for the patient with prolonged illness represents the end of one era and the beginning of another. Her very presence symbolizes the concern of the community in general, and the medical profession in particular, with the patient as a whole. As her services have grown in quality and depth, they have in turn deepened the total quality of care of patients whose problems cannot be dispelled through the scientific magic of antibiotics. The whole change in the concept of care for this group is perhaps best illustrated by the gradual abandoning of the term "chronic illness" with its implication of hopelessness and despair and the adoption of

the more descriptive and more dynamic term "prolonged illness." Whereas the "chronic" patient entered an institution
to die, the patient with prolonged illness nowadays enters a
hospital to receive needed treatment and, eventually, to leave
its confines.

While it is true that the dramatic achievements of medical
science in the conquest of many acute illnesses during the
past century have, as yet, not been duplicated in the field of
prolonged illness, some progress, nevertheless, has been
made. Not so long ago a diagnosis of diabetes meant that the
patient was condemned to early death or lifelong invalidism.
Now, many patients suffering from diabetes are not only able
to function with the aid of insulin, but to lead productive,
satisfying lives with a feeling of considerable comfort and
well-being. The progress made is well illustrated by the
slogan adopted by a group of diabetics: "Take the 'die' out of
diabetes."

This changing concept has brought with it the conviction
that our present-day facilities for caring for the patient with
prolonged illness lag far behind the medical and social
knowledge at our disposal. Most of the available facilities,
scant as they are, are relics of the past when our concept of
the untreatability of the "chronic" patient influenced the
provisions made for his care.

Even today, the very fact that in some instances a separate
hospital for such patients is still considered necessary throws
light on the philosophy behind its existence. It indicates that
the patient with prolonged illness is still viewed as someone
separate from, and by implication different from, other sick
people, requiring a different kind of help in a different kind
of institution.

Those most closely in contact with the problem of prolonged illness view the "chronic disease hospital" as an anachronism. They contend that, even if the level of care rendered is on a par with that given by the general hospital, special institutions should not be perpetuated, since the separation between "acute" and "chronic" is fading away and only appears nowadays as a "survival of the prescientific era." [1]

A sound program of medical care for the future has been formulated in this way:

The care of the acute (short-term) patient and the care of the chronic (long-term) patient should be integrated in the general hospital on a continuing basis as long as the need for a hospital bed can be proved; the care of all others should be provided in their homes, or in the equivalent of their homes, by an extramural hospital program, equal in service to the intramural hospital program. [2]

In order to realize the kind of integration that such a program suggests, it is necessary that the community gain a better understanding of what prolonged illness means in human terms. Who is the patient with prolonged illness? What are his individual problems? How do they affect him, his family, and his community? What kind of help does he need? How can it best be offered him? How can we use our present-day facilities in order to build for the future? What needs to be added to assure a well-rounded medical-social program? Drawing on experience with a group of patients suffering from prolonged illness, this book is devoted to an exploration of these questions in the conviction that once the full extent and manifold ramifications of the problem are fully appreciated, necessary provisions will be made to lessen the burden on those afflicted.

[1] Bluestone, "A Program for Prolonged Illness," p. 46.
[2] Bluestone, "Long-Term Illness in Modern Society," p. 1052.

3

THE EXTENT OF
THE PROBLEM

To ENCOMPASS the full implication of the effects of prolonged illness in all its aspects we need to know, first of all,
the extent of the problem. How many in our world today are
victims of prolonged illness? Are there more of these patients
today than there were a few generations ago? What are the
factors responsible for the increase, if any? Who are the
patients? Does such illness strike one sex more frequently
than the other, one age more often than another? Is it
influenced by economic status? How does such illness affect
the patient's ability to maintain his independent economic
status? What is the effect on the patient's family? What is the
cost to the community?

PAUCITY OF RELIABLE DATA

In the continued absence of systematic, comprehensive reporting answers to such questions are not easily available. A
survey of hospitals, sanatoria, and various other institutions
may give us some indication of the number of ill persons who
are no longer able to maintain themselves in the community.
Such figures, however, would account for only a small proportion of the total. Many patients with prolonged illness,
either partially or wholly disabled, remain in the community
sometimes by choice, sometimes because of lack of suitable
facilities. Still others, particularly in the early stages of their
illness, may even be functioning in their usual, normal way

with but occasional episodes of indisposition and interruption of normal routine.

The impression gained by those who come into contact with prolonged illness in their day-by-day observations—doctors, nurses, social workers—is that prolonged illness is widespread, that it affects all strata of the population without regard to age, sex, or economic status, and that it exacts a heavy toll in human suffering, directly over the area surrounding the patient, and indirectly over a much wider area.

The designation "prolonged" is applicable to the illness not only because, once established, it is of long duration but because the onset is often protracted and insidious. While acute illness has, generally speaking, a well-defined, sudden, dramatic onset, the onset of prolonged illness is usually gradual, slow, almost imperceptible, with little significance attached to early symptoms. In other instances, prolonged illness occurs as a sequela of acute illness. The victim of a prolonged illness in its early stages may recognize only his reduced work capacity, fatigue, and general malaise. These symptoms may be attributed to "that extra drink I took last night" or "the pickle I should not have eaten" or "the sleep I failed to get." Often considered too trifling to bring to the attention of a physician, these symptoms may be the warning and beginning of a disease process which medicine dignifies in its final stages with the name "prolonged illness." Until recently, few of these early manifestations came to the attention of the medical practitioner, and even when a doctor was consulted, their significance, in many instances, was not grasped. When the discomfort caused by the illness finally became sufficiently severe to force the victim to seek active medical attention, the disease process was well advanced and the possibility for arresting it slim. As a result, the medical profession heretofore sought acute rather than prolonged illness for study because in the latter case the disease was advanced, the damage done seemed irreversible, and the only solution appeared to be "custodial" or "terminal" care— meaning, in effect, nonmedical care.

It is only within recent years that attention has been drawn to prolonged illness as a public health problem of the first magnitude. We are witnessing a growing concern about its extent and its implications for world progress and a beginning attempt to study the problem in all its aspects.

The most complete data on the extent and significance of prolonged illness on a national level are those found in the National Health Survey on Chronic Conditions and Activity Limitation. This study was conducted during a two-year period, from July, 1961, to June, 1963, for the purpose of determining the prevalence of certain chronic conditions and the limitations in activity these imposed. As defined in the report, limitation of activity "refers not only to the major activity of the person (his ability to work, keep house, or engage in school or preschool activities) but also to his other pursuits, such as participation in recreational, civic, and similar activities." [1]

The study is based on information collected by means of household interviews and covered some 80,000 households containing 259,000 persons. The material included information about the civilian, noninstitutional population as regards sex, age, race, marital status, family income, usual activity status, and duration of bed disability in a year. When the results were analyzed, estimates were made as to the prevalence of chronic illness in the country as a whole and the resulting activity limitation.

The report emphasizes certain limitations inherent in the study. It points out that "since the estimates are based on a sample, they will differ somewhat from the figures that would

[1] U.S. Public Health Service, *Chronic Conditions and Activity Limitation*, p. 3. All statistics cited in this chapter, unless otherwise indicated, are taken from this study.

have been obtained if a complete census had been taken.
. . . As in any survey, the results are also subject to measure-
ment error. . . . There are limitations to the accuracy of
diagnostic and other information collected in household
interviews. For diagnostic information, the household re-
spondent can, at best, pass on to the interviewer only the
information the physician has given the family. For conditions not medically attended, diagnostic information is often
no more than a description of symptoms." [2]

It is well known that such a description may not give an
accurate picture of the condition. Furthermore, the importance of symptoms is frequently not recognized until the
disease process has been active for some time. It is, therefore,
reasonable to assume that early undiagnosed manifestations
were probably not reported in a substantial proportion of
cases. Even in some advanced cases, it is conceivable that the
informant was not aware that he had a pathological condition, particularly if the condition was not a disabling one.
The records of insurance companies supply ample testimony
to the fact that many people are unaware of having a serious
prolonged illness and discover it only during the routine
physical examination which the insuring company requires
of an applicant.

It must also be borne in mind that this survey embraces
but part of the chronically ill since it is concerned only with
the noninstitutional population. To this number must be
added not only the 800,000 older people in institutions, as
estimated by the President's Council on Aging,[3] but also the
unknown number of younger people who were in institutions at that time.

Impressive as these figures are, they do not tell the whole
story, for chronic conditions are not confined to physical
ailments. In another study conducted by the U.S. Public

[2] Ibid., p. 13.
[3] President's Council on Aging, The Older American, p. 12.

Health Service,[4] an estimate was made of the number of patients fifteen years of age and over in the 414 long-stay mental hospitals. This study conducted in April-June of 1963 found that there were approximately 558,000 patients in these institutions, which included hospitals under federal, state, and county as well as nongovernmental auspices. This number did not include, however, patients in maximum security wards and children's wards in these hospitals, nor those in mental hospitals serving children only.

To this number of hospital patients must be added the large though undetermined number of patients suffering from prolonged mental ailments who remain outside institutions.

The long-term nature of mental illness can be judged by the fact that, according to the Public Health Survey, 40 percent of all patients had been in the hospital 10 years or longer, an additional 14 percent had been confined for a period of between 5 and 9 years, 23 percent between one and 4 years, and the remainder for less than one year. The average length of stay following the last admission was 10.6 years.[5]

In view of the various limitations in both studies, their findings are the more significant in emphasizing the extent and widespread effect of prolonged illness.

Let us look at these findings.

ESTIMATED EXTENT OF THE PROBLEM

On the basis of the study on chronic conditions and activity limitation, it is estimated that some 80.3 million persons, or 44.1 percent of the civilian noninstitutional population, were suffering from one or more chronic diseases or impairment. Of these, about 22.2 million were limited in their activities to some degree.

[4] U.S. Public Health Service, *Characteristics of Patients in Mental Hospitals*, p. 3.
[5] *Ibid.*, p. 6.

Six majors categories of conditions were found to be responsible for the limitations, namely, heart ailments, arthritis and rheumatism, mental and nervous conditions, impairment of back and spine, impairment of lower extremities and hips, and hypertension without heart involvement.

INCREASE IN THE NUMBER OF PATIENTS
WITH PROLONGED ILLNESS

Not only is the number of people with prolonged illness large, but available figures support the general impression that it is constantly on the increase. This may be accounted for, at least in part, as being due to: (*a*) longevity; (*b*) our greater awareness of its early manifestations; (*c*) the more extensive use of medical attention in the beginning stages; and (*d*) more highly developed medical diagnostic skills.

We are living in a medically sophisticated age. Schools, newspapers, popular magazines, are health conscious. Such national agencies as the American Heart Association, Inc., the National Foundation, the National Tuberculosis Association, the American Cancer Society, Inc., and others, as well as the insurance companies are waging intensive educational campaigns designed to acquaint the general public with the symptoms of various illnesses in order to encourage the quest for early medical care. The very fact that these agencies carry on yearly drives for funds serves to keep people aware of the illnesses these agencies are organized to combat. By their emphasis on the significance of apparently minor symptoms, they have motivated people to bring their medical needs, no matter how slight the complaint may appear to be, to the attention of a physician. As a result of this emphasis on health, more and more people are turning to physicians, clinics, and hospitals for periodic check-ups, and for help before instead of after the fact. Consequently, the presumably unimportant symptoms, which in the past were neglected, are brought to the attention of the physician earlier.

The physician on his part, because of the greater knowledge now at his disposal, is in a better position to recognize and deal with many illnesses which formerly went undiagnosed. Thus medicine is in a position not only to see incipient manifestations of disease, but to identify and treat as disease entities conditions which at one time were overlooked because of medical inadequacy.

EFFECT OF ADVANCES IN MEDICAL SCIENCE

The primary reason for the increase in the number of patients suffering from known prolonged illness stems from the very advances made by medical science. These have brought about a general decrease in the incidence and fatal outcome of communicable diseases. Through sanitation, pasteurization, inoculation, and other procedures, we have witnessed the virtual elimination of epidemics. The development of new scientific techniques, antibiotics, the sulfa drugs, and chemotherapy in general have made possible a sharp reduction in the fatal outcome of such acute illnesses as pneumonia, appendicitis, mastoiditis, typhoid fever, and malaria, which in the past have been responsible for many deaths and often developed into chronic conditions. Communicable diseases of childhood and youth have been conquered to a large extent. As so graphically described by Geddes Smith:

The black plague that ravaged Europe is all but gone. The yellow fever that made men pray for winter is all but gone. The malignant choking death that struck children is all but gone. Purging fevers no longer haunt the waters that cities drink. Cheeks that would once have been pitted with smallpox are smooth and fresh. Men and women die old.[6]

EFFECT OF CHANGES IN AGE DISTRIBUTION

By saving innumerable young lives, by enabling men and women to live longer, medical advances have added many potential candidates for the so-called "degenerative" and

6 Smith, p. 1.

"malignant" diseases of maturity and old age. In fact, the age distribution of the entire population has been changed as a result of these medical advances. According to figures compiled in the National Council on the Aging, "of the total population today [1964], one person out of every 11 is past 65, in comparison to only one in 25 at the turn of the century." [7] The number of persons over 65 had risen to 19 million by July 1, 1966, according to figures released by the Social Security Administration, and it was estimated by the National Council on the Aging that this number will probably rise to over 25 million by 1985. [8]

The change in population trends and the increase in the number of older people in our midst brings us face to face with the realization that we are living in an era of an aging population. Consequently, the problems created by prolonged illness with their emotional, economic, and social ravages are assuming ever greater proportions. This means not only that more people will be subject to the progressive degenerative and malignant diseases prevalent among those of middle age or older, but that these diseases will persist over long periods of time. While prolonged illness is not exclusively, or even primarily, confined to old age, the incidence increases with aging. Not only is prolonged illness more prevalent among the older age groups, but the social problems created by chronicity are more pronounced. The older the patient, the more complicated is his medical and eventually his social history; the higher the incidence of complicating illnesses, the scantier his recuperative powers and the longer the period during which active medical care is imperative.

Important as are the degenerative diseases of the old, and in spite of the existing tendency to lump the aged and the "chronics" so that they become almost synonymous in the

[7] *Background Facts on the Income of Older People,* p. 1.
[8] *Ibid.*

minds of many people, we must remember that the greatest threat to communal well-being lies in the fact that prolonged illness strikes all age groups, the young as well as the old. For instance, the National Health Survey indicates that 12,856,000 persons under 17 years of age are afflicted with one or more chronic conditions. It is difficult to determine the diagnostic groupings of these younger patients, for in the distribution by diagnosis, those under 17 years of age are included with all persons under 45. Nor does the study of patients in mental hospitals give the number of patients in the younger age category separately; rather they are grouped together with all patients under 44 years of age.

No diagnostic categories are given for the patients in mental hospitals. They are considered in relation to their ambulation, continence, awareness of surroundings, hearing ability, and vision. Nor are diagnoses given for the physically incapacitated patients. It is known however, that polio, the killer and maimer of children in the past, is now on the decline. So is tuberculosis. While cancer and diabetes are not so frequent among children as they are among adults, they nevertheless exist. Similarly, while rheumatic fever with its sequelae of damaged hearts and kidneys is found less often than it was in the past, it still occurs, and the resulting damage and impairment are long term in nature. And we need only mention the prevalence of cerebral palsy, cardiac conditions, and various orthopedic and neuromuscular diseases in children to realize how susceptible the young may be to the ravages of prolonged illness and its residual effects.

According to the National Health Survey the proportion of persons with one or more chronic physical conditions increases with age. Thus, 19.9 percent were persons under 17 years of age; 47.5 percent were between 17 and 44 years old; 64.1 percent were between 45 and 64; and 81.0 percent were over 64. While the age groupings, as here given, make it impossible to determine the percentage of those with prolonged illness who were in the productive years of life, it is evident that well over two thirds fall within this category.

The advances in medical science, through the arrest of the disease process and the conquest of many of the ailments which previously proved fatal at an early stage, have succeeded in keeping alive many of these younger victims of prolonged illness, however handicapped. The very fact that they live longer with the residual aspects of their illness creates numerous social problems for them, their families, and the community. This phenomenon is indeed having the effect of drawing the medical profession and the profession of social work closer to each other.

THE EFFECT OF PROLONGED ILLNESS ON EVERYDAY LIVING

It is obvious from the figures here quoted that prolonged illness is a problem in every stage of life and that it strikes indiscriminately. Translated into human terms, it is a problem of the school child who is subject to rheumatic fever, convulsive disorders, poliomyelitis, even malignant neoplasms. It is a problem of the housewife who is a likely target for malignant tumors and circulatory disorders. The businessman is particularly receptive to such diverse illnesses as ulcers of the digestive tract and Buerger's disease. The laborer is a frequent victim of arthritis, tuberculosis, and cardiovascular disease. The doctor too fears the coronary attack for himself.

Because of the breadth of its coverage, prolonged illness affects school adjustment, choice of employment, continuity of work, professional and social achievement, marriage, and family life generally. In short, every aspect of living is influenced by the illness, which interferes with the aims, goals, and ambitions people set for themselves, frequently putting an end to all that for them makes life worth living.

Behind the men and women whose illnesses are publicized

lies the great mass of humanity whose struggle with their handicaps goes more or less unnoticed. The extent of the suffering that illness creates can be appreciated only if one looks at hospital charts, the records of private physicians, and among the cases of social agencies. Neither the medical profession nor social agencies, however, feel the full impact of prolonged illness except, perhaps, in its final stages. In the final analysis, the magnitude and far-reaching significance of the problems it creates are felt by the patient himself and those who are most closely associated with him—his family. Initially, the illness may manifest itself only in a day lost from school or work, irritability over a bridge hand one fails to make, or a spanking motivated more by mother's headache than Johnny's naughtiness. As the disease progresses, however, these minor disturbances may come to mean much more. It is the cumulative effect of days lost, of constant irritability and disrupted family harmony, of discomfort, pain, and suffering that makes prolonged illness so devastating in human terms.

LOSS OF PRODUCTIVITY

Though no accurate count of days lost from work is possible, this loss is undoubtedly an important factor since so many of those afflicted are in the productive years of life. Any illness necessarily interferes with an individual's productive capacity. In the case of an acutely ill patient, the period of enforced idleness is usually limited and often endurable, economically and otherwise. Not so in prolonged illness. Not only is the period of hospitalization and of medical care generally longer, but, in addition, the illness frequently leaves in its wake either partial or total incapacity. Thus, the National Health Survey found that almost one fourth of all persons suffering from one or more chronic conditions were limited in their activity to a greater or lesser degree. Of these, over 4.1 million persons were unable to carry on their major activity; 12 million more were limited in the amount and kind of major activity they were able to perform, and an additional 6.1 million were limited although not in their major activity.

The large and ever increasing number of persons 65 years of age and over, as well as the incidence of prolonged illness among them, and the variety of problems it creates, tend at times to obscure the incidence and importance of prolonged illness and its sequelae among younger people. And yet, according to the survey estimates, there were over 14 million people under 65 years of age so afflicted as to be limited in activity. This number would be considerably larger if those confined to institutions were included.

The figures indicate that for a substantial number of those studied, such limitation of activity would entail reduction in productive employment and would result in serious consequences for the economy of the group. It means curtailment of income, disappearance of savings, indebtedness, lowering of living standards, strains and stresses of all kinds. Later we shall discuss how this may affect the individual patient and his family. Here we are concerned primarily with the overall picture.

PROLONGED ILLNESS AND POVERTY: THE VICIOUS CIRCLE

Family income has a significant bearing on the presence or absence of chronic conditions and activity limitation of the individuals in the family, according to the National Health Survey. In fact, it states that "there is an inverse relationship . . . . between the amount of family income and the proportion of chronic disease and impairment and associated limitation of activity." [9]

This does not come as a surprise. While it may not always be possible to determine which is cause and which is effect, it

[9] U.S. Public Health Service, *Chronic Conditions and Activity Limitations*, p. 8.

has long been recognized that prolonged illness and poverty pursue each other, and eventually go hand in hand.

The relation of some forms of prolonged illness to poor economic conditions is well known, such as the relation of tuberculosis to low standards of living, overwork, overcrowding; the effects of poor diet have been pointed out over and over again and need no further elaboration. Similarly, the tendency to rheumatic fever with its sequela, rheumatic heart disease, is increased by poverty, poor diet, overcrowding, and the unhygienic surroundings frequently found among low-income groups.

In addition, poor financial circumstances often mean delayed medical attention or the total lack of it at the onset of an acute illness. Any disease which begins as an acute illness can become chronic in time. Acute bronchitis, for example, is the potential form of chronic bronchitis; acute appendicitis may develop into chronic appendicitis; an acute rheumatic flare-up may mean the onset of rheumatoid arthritis. Adequate medical attention at the very beginning and throughout the acute episode is often the only means of preventing an acute illness from developing into a prolonged illness. Unfortunately, only too frequently such medical care is not easily available to people in the low-income group.

Even when medical facilities are available, financial pressures may interfere with the carrying out of the physician's recommendations. A special diet which may be an essential form of treatment may prove prohibitive in cost. The need to work in order to live may make it impossible to adhere to the doctor's recommendation for a prolonged rest which would arrest the spread of the disease, or prevent a recurrence. Again, tuberculosis is a good illustration. In its early stages, the disease can be controlled in most instances, provided complete rest and adequate treatment are secured. One cannot help but wonder how many patients in the low economic group, driven by the necessity to earn a living, ignore this recommendation until the ravages created by an advanced stage of the disease leave them no choice. Similarly, in cardiac ailments, the largest single group in the classification of prolonged illnesses and so often resulting in permanent handicap, lack of early diagnosis, the inability to secure the proper rest, and the need to continue working even though it be injurious are important factors in aggravating the condition to a point where it becomes irreversible and permanently incapacitating.

The foregoing discussion clearly indicates that the development of prolonged illness may be influenced or aggravated by poor economic conditions; and the presence of such illness further depresses the economic status by interfering with earning capacity, while the cost of necessary medical care saps available resources. The net result is that the overwhelming burden of the cost of prolonged illness, with the frequently permanent invalidism which it causes, falls upon the group least able to bear it. The following statement summarizes the entire situation succinctly: "These patients are located within a vicious circle, for poverty aggravates chronic disease and chronic disease will pauperize a patient if it keeps up long enough, which is often the case." [10]

Furthermore, our increased awareness of the importance of the social and emotional components in illness does not allow us to overlook the effect of this vicious circle upon the patient's ability to respond to treatment when it is finally secured. All too frequently, curtailment of earnings and worry over its effect upon those dependent upon him are potent factors which influence adversely the progress of the patient even when he is given the best possible medical attention.

THE MORTALITY RATE

The mortality rate is another important indication of the ravages of prolonged illness. It is normally to be expected that in an aging population the total death rate from such

[10] Bluestone, "The Chronic Has a Claim," p. 68.

illness will be on the increase. With the better control of infectious and acute illness, all authorities agree that we are witnessing a shift from acute to prolonged disease as a major cause of death.

According to a study conducted by the Public Health Service, based on data secured from a "survey of places which provided care in the last year of life to a sample of persons who died in 1961 the largest number of deaths are caused by cardiovascular diseases, cancer, and vascular lesions affecting the central nervous system." [11]

These figures do not tell the whole story. As we think of prolonged illness and its implications, of what it means to ever increasing numbers of people, it is important to remember that the limitations of the National Health Survey and other studies result in an underestimation rather than an overestimation of the full extent of the problem. If all the facts were available, we would then have the full impact of a problem wide in its distribution, affecting all parts of the population, costly in terms of disability, loss of productivity, and mortality—costly, above all else, in human suffering and deprivation.

On the basis of these admittedly low estimates, we have over 80 million noninstitutional people in the United States suffering from some chronic disease or impairment. Of these, over 22 million, in addition to almost 600,000 in mental hospitals, as well as uncounted thousands in the community, are limited in their activities to some degree; over one half of them are under 65 years of age.

These are staggering figures indeed, and their very magnitude may obscure the suffering and burden imposed on the individual and his family. For he who gets sick is more than a statistical figure. He is a human being. He is suffering; he is doubting; he is afraid. How can we help him combat anxie-

[11] U.S. Public Health Service, *Hospitalization in the Last Years of Life,* p. 17.

ties and fears which so frequently stand in the way of his utilizing to the utmost the medical and social facilities available for his care? How can we help him achieve his maximum recovery and to accept this maximum no matter how short it falls of his own goals? What other goals can we substitute for those he has to give up? What can we do to enhance his feeling that he is a functioning, useful member of society in spite of his limitations?

If we are to become fully aware of the extent of the problem, more accurate and up-to-date studies are essential. The answers to the questions of what it means to the individual patient who is sick and what can be done to help him, will have to come through other sources, however. These can be supplied only through the development of a philosophy which stresses interest in the person who is sick, his dignity and worth as an individual, and embraces not only the treatment of a disease, but that of the whole person, no matter to what point the disease may have progressed.

4

RAVAGES OF
PROLONGED ILLNESS

THE OVERWHELMING MAGNITUDE of prolonged illness tends to point up its significance in human terms, and its meaning to the particular patient and his family. To appreciate its full impact—the suffering and deprivation it inflicts and the upheavals it creates—let us look for a moment not at the staggering number of over 80 million chronic sufferers, but at some individual case histories.

THE MEANING OF ILLNESS
TO THE PATIENT

Here are seven entries taken from the notebook of the social worker who sees each applicant for admission to her hospital. Each one of these case histories tells a story that may well be repeated among our friends and neighbors, in the home of our grocery clerk, our family doctor, our children's teacher, or the boy who delivers the morning paper. They are of importance to all of us, if we are to appreciate the full significance of prolonged illness and its implications.

Let us see what these entries tell us.

The first patient who entered the worker's office one morning was Mr. F., 41 years old; he told the worker that he had an ulcer of the right foot. Mr. F. worked as a laboratory technician earning $94 per week but had been unemployed for the past seven weeks. He had exhausted his unemployment insurance benefits, and his sick benefits had been used up during previous hospitalizations. His wife worked in the same hospital and earned $55 per week. A daughter of 14 attended school.

At the time he applied for admission and gave the factual data for his application form, we could only hazard a guess as to what this hospitalization meant to him. He had been ill on and off for many years and had been hospitalized several times. This, in itself, gave us some idea of the discouragement with which he must be facing yet another hospitalization; for each relapse, each new hospitalization, inevitably undermines the patient's faith in his eventual recovery. Even when his symptoms subside and he is apparently feeling better, the fear of recurrence becomes as much a threat as the reality of the illness itself.

Sick and unemployment benefits having been exhausted, and with diminishing faith in his ability to return to work, to hold a job, Mr. F. was haunted by the specter of financial difficulties. With their combined earnings, Mr. F. and his wife were able to maintain a decent standard of living. What would happen to this standard with the income cut in half? How long would he remain unemployed? Suppose he never could return to normal employment again—what would be the effect on his daughter? Would she have to give up schooling as soon as she was of age in order to supplement the family income? Under these circumstances, how patient could this man be in following out the medical recommendation for prolonged treatment and subsequent rest? Would his faith in medical treatment continue, or would he, under pressure of economic conditions and worry about his family, return to work sooner than advisable, only to face another exacerbation of his illness and yet another hospitalization?

Next came Miss Z. She was 26 years old and was being transferred from a city hospital, with a diagnosis of rheumatic heart disease. Illness struck two years ago. At that time she was forced to give up her job as a glovemaker and enter a city hospital. She had no one to whom she could turn for help; her mother was dead, her father estranged from the family for many years; two brothers were living in furnished rooms, barely able to make ends meet. At the time of her admission to the city hospital she had to give up her small apartment, which represented the only home she knew. The demands of the illness thus superseded all the hopes and wishes any young girl might have for herself.

As she faced another hospitalization, what could her outlook be for the future? Should she fail to notice any appreciable improvement as a result of medical treatment, the realization must gradually come that her chances for returning to her former employment were diminishing. Eventually, she might be permanently handicapped. As we saw her total problem, we could but wonder at the reservoirs of hope and will to live which sustained her and gave her the strength necessary to continue the fight.

For Mr. L., illness caused yet another kind of dislocation, affecting not only himself, but his wife and his children as well. A tailor by trade, he had been in and out of hospitals for the past two years. Now, at the age of 55, he was being admitted with a diagnosis of destructive lesion of the right hip. During his illness, his wife had to shoulder the greater part of the burden since he was able to work only sporadically. She found employment as a finisher in the clothing industry and earned $80 per week. Their 18-year-old daughter abandoned her plans for further education and left school to work as a clerk in order to help provide necessities for the family and the few extras Mr. L.'s illness demanded; a 15-year-old son attended high school.

Two years is a long time to be sick and unemployed. To Mr. L.'s worry about his condition was added the strain of watching his wife go to work and assume the major responsibility of maintaining the family. As the patient was faced with still another hospitalization, concern about his son's future preyed on his mind. Would his son too have to leave school and swell the ranks of unskilled workers—the group most susceptible to job-market fluctuations? Mr. L. had dreamed of another future for his children and now, helpless, he must see his dreams shattered by his illness.

Not only his immediate family, but Mr. C.'s partner as well felt the effects of Mr. C.'s illness. The few facts gleaned about Mr. C. at the point of admission indicated the disruption of independent living created by prolonged illness. At the age of 50 he was being hospitalized with a diagnosis of cancer of the stomach. He had been working as a hat cleaner in partnership with another man. For the past year he had been irregular in his attendance at the store, missing a day now and then because of ill health. For the past two months, as his condition became worse, he had not been able to attend to the business, and his partner had to employ a helper. Consequently, Mr. C. was left entirely without income. Mrs. C., at 44, was forced to look for employment. She had never worked, had no particular skills, and, under the circumstances, whatever work she might be able to obtain would be of an unskilled nature and poorly paid. A daughter of 14 attended high school. In addition to the discomfort and pain of the illness this patient had to witness the defeat of his plans for himself and his family.

And what of the defeat that Mr. E. was suffering? At 74 he was finally forced to give in to the ravages of pulmonary tuberculosis, an illness of several years' duration. Never a rich man, he had nevertheless managed by working as a butcher to save enough money to carry him through several years of unemployment. Anxiously he watched his meager savings dwindling and now he had only $70 left, he told the social worker. His wife had died eight years ago. There were no children. We could only speculate on the economies he had had to practice in order to maintain his independence for so long a period. His savings, to him, represented security. What faced him now at 74, ill with only $70 and no family on whom he could lean?

Mr. Y., 45 years old, was being admitted with a diagnosis of prosacral abscess, cancer of the stomach. He had been ill for three years. His 34-year-old wife took care of the home and their 7½-year-old son. A little over three years ago Mr. Y. had purchased a partnership in a liquor store with money borrowed from his wife's relatives. His drawing account never exceeded $50 to $60 a week, barely enough to maintain his family and certainly not enough for him to be able to save or to repay the loan.

At first glance, Mr. Y.'s financial situation might have appeared a little brighter than that of some of the other patients we have been discussing. He had a small independent business, and his wife, who helped him before his illness, would be able to carry on so that their income would continue. But what about the child? How much attention would the mother be able to give him, tied as she would be to the business? Would the small retail store become the child's home and the sidewalk his playground? What about the money borrowed from relatives? What were the chances of its being repaid? And what would happen to the family relationships when the loan was not repaid, when it became apparent that it could never be repaid?

Mrs. M., age 33, was suffering from a pituitary adenoma and rheumatic heart disease. She had been ill for several years, had been receiving sporadic medical attention without much benefit, and was finally told she must be hospitalized. As a matter of fact, the doctor had urged hospitalization long ago, but she could not make up her mind to follow his advice. She did not know what to do about the children. She could not leave them alone. The oldest of the five children was 13, the youngest 5. They needed attention and supervision. Her husband, busy with his job as order clerk in a food company, could not give them the care they needed.

Mrs. M.'s illness was not only serious in its immediate implications but was likely to leave her with a permanent incapacity. The impact would be felt not only by her, but also by her 37-year-old husband left to cope with five children. What plans could be made for these children? On his salary it would be almost impossible to secure competent help in the home. Would it be necessary to break up the home, even if only temporarily? Or would an undue share of the burden fall upon the 13-year-old, hardly old enough to carry it?

When Mrs. M. is finished with hospital treatment and is ready to return home, the residual handicap left by the illness may prevent her from resuming full responsibility for the household. Whatever plans are made to maintain the family unit must not only take into consideration the existing emergency, but must be projected into the future. The whole structure of family life is being threatened, and radical changes may have to be made.

These are but a few situations taken at random on one single day. In this small series we have illustrations of some of the manifold implications of prolonged illness as they affect the patient and his family. Multiply these by the number of people with prolonged illness in the world today, and we have not only a gigantic social problem but one with all-pervading medical, emotional, and economic implications. Discouragement, fear of recurrence, defeat of plans and hopes for the future, economic insecurity, lowering of standards, exhaustion of savings, mounting debts, recognition of the ever diminishing hope for the future, all these are frequent concomitants of prolonged illness.

By the time these patients had left the hospital, a great deal more was known about each of them, and the social worker had occasion to help them not only with their medical problems, but with many others which their illnesses brought in their wake. At the time of a patient's admission we can only draw upon our accumulated experience and on the basis of that experience surmise what these problems are, what the patient may have to face, and what help he may need.

Loss of employment, indebtedness, the breaking up of the home, discomfort and pain—these are terms with which we are all familiar. At one time or another we may have seen any one of them or a combination, or all. Most acute illnesses carry with them pain and discomfort. The sudden change of an individual from an independent, normally functioning, productive member of society to a dependent, helpless invalid is familiar to us. We are all aware of the social implications of such a transition. Difficult as these adjustments are, the acutely ill patient can usually derive comfort and strength in meeting them, aware of their temporary nature and conscious of his gradual improvement.

Unlike the acutely ill patient, the one with prolonged ill-ness is depressed by his body's failure to respond to therapy. When his condition does not improve, doubt creeps in and finally becomes his constant companion. Fear, anxiety, and often panic gnaw at his vitals. What if he will never be able to return to work? How long will his savings hold out? How soon will his friends and relatives "write him off"? Wasn't Aunt Jane less approachable about money this week than she was four weeks ago?

Illness not only interrupts the ordinary pattern of living, it affects the person's feelings about himself. Something hap-pens to the ego of the person who feels that his customary way of coping with life is slipping from him. It is one thing to ask for a loan with the firm belief that in a week or a month, or even a year, he can pay it back; it is quite another to ask for a loan when the request carries with it no personal conviction of ability to repay. Does the lender share your doubt? If he does, how long will he continue to lend to you, if at all? How long will it be before he recognizes the true state of affairs? And when this happens, what will it do to the confidence and trust of a friendship built up through many years of giving and taking? It is one thing to ask Aunt Mary to take the children for a few weeks till you get your strength back; it is quite another when time passes, the weeks succeed one another, and both you and she begin to question how long the "few weeks" will be. As months pass, and you are still unable to care for the children, will Aunt Mary continue to help? If not, what other arrangements can be made? Will they have to be shifted from one relative's home to another? Will they have to go to an institution?

What happens to these children? Too young to appreciate the real reason for the arrangements, do they feel that they are being "sent away," pushed out of the home, that they no longer "belong"? Do they begin to doubt the love of the par-ent who puts them into someone else's home and cannot visit them? When the time comes for them to return, will they want to come back to a mother or a father who had "abandoned" them, had not come to visit? What will it mean to them to be in the home with a parent who is in almost constant pain, who cannot work, and who must ask them for help with the very details of living with which parents should help their children? Even if they want to do it, should they be asked to make the sacrifices?

We recall Mr. B., a former prize fighter who at the age of 32 was stricken with amyotrophic lateral sclerosis, a degenerative neurological illness. When he came to the clinic he was always accompanied by his 7-year-old son, who helped him in and out of the cab, buttoned his overcoat, tied his shoes. To all outward appearances, here was the picture of a perfect father-son relationship—companionship, helpfulness, love. It needed only one question from the social worker as to Mr. B.'s reaction to his dependence on his son to reveal what was hidden behind the positive picture and the emotional cost of maintaining it. All the hopelessness that Mr. B. felt about his illness, all the defeat, the despair, were centered in the fact that his son, whom he should be helping, was tying his shoes. How could he matter as a father, how could he advise, how could he discipline, when his son was making it possible for him to get the medical care he needed, seeing him in his weakness and his helplessness, not in his strength?

No one single illustration, or any group of illustrations, can convey what prolonged illness means to patients. What the patient's reaction will be, is determined in considerable measure by the patient himself, the kind of person he is, what he expects of life, what his goals and ambitions are. Into all of this go his past experiences and his reactions to them. The emotional response, so important in any illness, becomes even more important when the illness not merely demands a temporary readjustment, but cuts across the patient's established pattern of living and compels him to formulate a new way of life governed by the requirements of his particular disability. How the patient feels about his illness, how he reacts to it, what use he makes of it, and how he can use that part of himself which is not sick will determine his future and will help or hinder him in the process of building a new life.

For Mr. Jones, unable to face the real reason for his lack of success in a competitive world, a severe cardiac condition which removes him from competition may come as a release. For Mr. Smith, who sees his value to his family solely or primarily on the basis of his ability to provide well, the same cardiac condition may be catastrophic, since it robs him of this status. What each will make of his cardiac condition will depend on his past pattern of behavior. Each will use his illness as he has used other life experiences to meet emotional needs and to get satisfactions directly or indirectly.

Mr. Jones, relieved as he may be of the constant strain which the unequal competition imposed on him, may derive satisfaction through surrender to his illness, or he may be induced with help to seek other satisfactions. Or, overcome by guilt, he may make the most of his illness, even reacting in an exaggerated way to his symptoms as if to demonstrate to himself, as well as to others, that his illness makes it impossible to expect anything of him. On the other hand, Mr. Smith, keenly aware of his loss of status, may, despite his doctor's recommendations, continue his usual pattern of living, actually committing slow suicide in the process. Or, given skilled help, he may come to see himself as a useful member of society even though his value be measured in terms other than financial success.

We could go on indefinitely in our speculations, for the reactions of different individuals to their illnesses are as different as the individuals themselves, and will be determined by all the life factors which went into making them what they are. Regardless of how the patient is eventually able to use that part of himself which remains undamaged by the disease, he is forced to make compromises which may be difficult and with which he may need help The patient with prolonged illness has to accept his illness and its limitations, follow its commands, obey the code of behavior it prescribes, in order to be able to live with it, or else it may destroy him. Neither Mr. Jones nor Mr. Smith can continue to function at all unless he recognizes that he can no longer function as he did in the past, and that his only chance of meaningful survival lies in the surrender of at least part of himself to his illness. Implicit in such a surrender is the concept that he has to become dependent. This dependence is of several types: he is dependent on the physician who prescribes the treatment; on the treatment itself; on the demands the illness makes upon him, frequently involving a change in his entire pattern of living. Furthermore, he may have to accept a dependence on others in performing the daily tasks which he previously performed unaided. This manifold dependence is likely to create many conflicts, for throughout life the basic pattern of acquiring independence has been fostered and even forced upon him. To learn to give up an independence achieved at great cost may mean a struggle, or it may mean a giving in to a long-cherished but suppressed wish. In either event, it means that he will have to make an adjustment to a new way of life, set new goals for himself, and find new satisfactions. The need to enter a hospital is the symbol of this need for a different adjustment.

MEDICAL CARE AT THE
ONSET OF ILLNESS

It has been our experience that for most patients, admission to a hospital for prolonged illness represents not their first contact with medical care, but, more likely, the last resort in a series of visits to physicians, clinics, or other hospitals—the choice being determined more often by the patient's economic status and the stage to which his illness has progressed than by his preferences. To understand fully what the patient's reaction to entering a hospital is likely to be, it is necessary to know what preceded it. Let us consider what the patient's experiences might have been in the course of his search for medical help; for these experiences and the attitudes he has consequently developed will have a profound influence on the way in which he will approach hospitalization and, therefore, on his response to medical care.

MEDICAL CARE IN A CLINIC

In many instances, prolonged illness is insidious in onset. The early symptoms seem hardly to warrant the consideration of hospitalization. They may, however, seriously interfere with the patient's earning capacity. As a result, long before the illness has reached the stage where hospitalization is required, many patients find that they have exhausted their resources and must resort to whatever free medical facilities the community provides.

It is a well-known fact that many of these facilities—the independent clinics and outpatient departments of hospitals—are overcrowded, with long waiting lists for admission. This in itself is no negligible factor, either from the standpoint of loss of earning capacity or the effect it has on the progress of the medical condition for which help is being sought. What is even more important is the fact that overcrowding means long waits at the clinic as well as hurried and sometimes superficial examinations. The present-day practice of medicine and the high degree of its specialization often necessitate referral of the patient from one clinic to another, from one specialty to another, before all tests are taken and a diagnosis can be established. As the patient is referred from clinic to clinic, he is subjected not to one, but to a succession of waiting periods. These numerous visits are time-consuming and add to the total number of days lost from work and consequent loss of earnings. Since the clinic patient is, to begin with, the economically deprived patient, the financial burden of time lost falls upon those least able to bear it. Worry about loss of earnings often leads to an intensification of symptoms, followed by more clinic visits, while the disease progresses and its ravages become more pronounced.

What is equally important is the effect these numerous referrals and delays have upon the patient's feelings about himself. The patient whose symptoms persist and become more incapacitating, who does not understand the need for the referrals, begins to question what it all means. He fears not only that there may be something radically wrong with him, but, even more disquieting, that the doctors do not know what it is and can do little to help him. As a rule, the hurried, overburdened clinic physician has but little time to explain, interpret, reassure; and the patient is left to cope with his anxieties as best he can. He has no idea what the difficulty is, or what he can expect.

MEDICAL CARE BY A PRIVATE PHYSICIAN

The patient who can afford to consult a private physician is in a better situation. In the office of the private physician he has more of the doctor's undivided attention, since he can pay for it, and therefore more opportunity to discuss matters at leisure and to become involved in what is happening to him. There too, however, the specialization in the medical profession may make it necessary to send the patient to specialists for supplementary tests and procedures. The net result often is that even the patient who can afford private medical care initially may find that by the time all the tests and procedures have been completed, his depleted resources are no longer adequate to cover the prescribed treatment.

The personal relationship of confidence and trust which the patient develops with his physician, a relationhip seldom possible in a clinic, may help to carry the patient through this period of diagnosis without arousing an undue amount of uncertainty and fear. The very nature of the illness, however, often precludes the possibility of any appreciable amelioration. As time passes without tangible results, the patient may find it increasingly difficult to accept as an explanation the prolonged nature of his illness and the need for continued treatment. Losing faith in the physician and the treatment, the patient may shop around for medical advice. As he sees one doctor after another, as different methods of treatment are tried with little, if any, relief from symptoms, as the economic drain increases, and as the encouragement he receives becomes meaningless in view of the progress of the illness, the patient may lose faith in doctors, in treatment, and in his own capacity to recover. He may become so discouraged as to give up looking for medical help until forced to do so again by physical discomfort, or he may go on searching. In either case, a great deal of precious time may be lost during which the disease progresses and its ravages become irreversible.

FACING THE NECESSITY FOR HOSPITALIZATION

The character of the onset, the nature of the early symptoms, and the periods of remission, so frequent in prolonged illness, all tend to blind the victim to the insidious characteristics of the disease. A time comes, however, when the symptoms can no longer be ignored or ascribed to any particular external cause, when the progress of the illness, the discomfort and pain, the vain search for relief, slowly force upon the patient the realization that his illness will take a long time to cure and that no quick improvement can be expected.

No matter how protracted the illness, or how extensive the amount of medical attention, the necessity of entering a hospital almost invariably comes as a shock. While the patient may derive some degree of consolation from the hope that at last he will receive the concentrated medical attention he has been seeking for so long, other problems confront him, as serious in their implications as the medical problem itself.

The notes on each patient made by the social worker at the time of admission indicate all too clearly the multiplicity of social problems which hospitalization brings to the fore. Some of these problems are pressing in their urgency and clamor for an immediate solution, if they are not to interfere with the patient's ability to avail himself of the benefits hospitalization holds for him. If the present-day understanding of the interrelation between emotional tensions and somatic disturbances is to be translated into actual practice for the welfare of the patient, help with such problems as beset him must be made available to the patient from the moment of his first contact with the hospital and throughout his stay.

Let us consider some of the problems which confront the patient at the time of admission. First and foremost is the frightening strangeness of the hospital. As a result, almost without exception, every patient, whether adult or child, has questions as to what hospitalization will be like, how long it will last, and what he can expect from it. These factors, which are inherent in any hospitalization, assume particular significance when the patient enters a hospital devoted exclusively to "chronic" diseases. The feeling of the community that such a hospital is the last stopping place and that admission is a symbol of defeat and medical hopelessness influences the patient's thinking, and he may need help with the anxiety it engenders.

Not only fear, anxiety, and hopelessness, but practical considerations as well, play their part. The ever mounting cost of hospital care poses a problem for many patients. Confronted with the realization of the expense involved and unaware of the resources available to him in the community, the patient may decide that it is impossible for him to finance such care. It is not enough, however, merely to tell him of possible avenues of supplementation, for the humiliation of accepting public assistance may outweigh even his desire to receive medical help. As an illustration, let us consider Mr. Brown:

A tall, rather handsome gentleman, Mr. Brown walked down the long corridor to the social worker's office, confused and bewildered. He had been told to see the social worker but he was sure there was nothing she could do to help him. Now that he knew what hospital care would cost, he realized that it was way beyond his means. It was true that Dr. White had urged him to enter the hospital as soon as possible, but apparently his physician did not understand his financial situation.

Still perplexed and completely ill at ease, Mr. Brown found himself in the social worker's office. He began to talk—at first hesitantly, then more freely. He was amazed at the worker's simple acceptance of his financial problem as though it were nothing out of the ordinary, her genuine interest in what he was saying, the absence of prying or curiosity. He found himself speaking of his illness, his family, and with pride he showed the social worker photographs of his children which he always carried in his wallet.

He removed his coat, settled back in his chair, and without his quite knowing how it happened he and the social worker were discussing ways and means of dealing with his problem. He eagerly reached for the pencil and paper which the worker offered him, saying, "This makes me feel at home. I've always worked with facts and figures." They discussed the family's finances, how much money he had, what his essential expenses were, and what would be left for medical care. He added up his income and expenditures, and no matter how they figured, Mr. Brown could see no way to meet the deficit. Since his doctor felt that hospital care was essential, Mr. Brown thought he might borrow the money from friends. The social worker wondered how practical this would be since no one could say with certainty how long he would be in the hospital, nor when he would be able to repay the loan. Quite simply, the social worker suggested that the city could meet the difference between what he could pay the hospital and what the charges would actually be. Mr. Brown's first reaction was that he did not want "charity." He had worked hard all his life and was accustomed to a "pay-as-you-go existence." He could not allow himself to digress from this pattern of living. The social worker explained that this was not charity; as a resident of the city who had paid his taxes for a number of years Mr. Brown had a right to such assistance. This seemed to make sense. He had never thought of it in this light; perhaps she was right.

After the necessary arrangements were made and Mr. Brown was ready to leave, he asked the social worker whether he would have an opportunity to see her again. She assured him that he would—many questions might arise in his mind which he might wish to discuss. She was there to assist him in carrying out a medical program outlined by his doctor and to help him with any other problems which might confront him. As Mr. Brown left the office he thanked the social worker for her understanding. He was a little clearer in his own mind now, and it was reassuring to know there was someone with whom he could share his problem.

Serious as the difficulty of meeting the cost of medical care may be, there are numerous other problems which appear insurmountable and may influence adversely the patient's decision to enter a hospital. There is the dilemma facing the breadwinner whose family is left without means of support; or that confronting the woman who feels she cannot enter the hospital because she does not know how to plan for the care of her small children; or the old man who feels he cannot leave his ailing blind wife alone in the apartment; or the high school student who must prepare for his final examinations.

If these patients, and others like them, are to receive whatever benefits medical science can offer, they need assistance in handling such problems. The social worker who sees the patient at the time when he has to make his decision can aid in removing whatever obstacles stand in the way of securing adequate medical help. Even when the nature of the problems precludes the possibility of an immediate solution, the patient's feeling of insecurity is diminished by the realization that he is not facing these difficulties unaided and that he can count on the social worker, on her understanding and assistance.

What other social and emotional problems face the patient in the hospital, what help he might need, and how that help can be given in a total well-integrated approach to the patient will be discussed later, as we follow the patient in the hospital, as we stay with him throughout his hospital experience, and help him plan for his future when he is ready to leave the hospital and resume life in the community.

5

THE MEANING OF HOSPITALIZATION

With the passage of time, increasing numbers of patients have come to appreciate hospitalization as a means of securing a thorough diagnostic work-up and treatment during the early stages of illness. The modern hospital, embracing the various specialties, having at its disposal the most up-to-date scientific and technical equipment for diagnostic and therapeutic procedures, can study the patient's condition and arrive at a diagnosis without loss of time, energy, or money. Treatment can be instituted early, and the disease can be arrested before it is too late.

THE PATIENT'S REACTION
TO HOSPITALIZATION

Unfortunately, however, many people still regard hospitalization with misgiving and apprehension. There are several reasons to account for the fact that they accept hospitalization only when an acute onset of symptoms forces them to do so, and often only after other means have failed. Primary among these reasons is the popular concept of the meaning of hospitalization and the fear of it. For many years, being hospitalized meant that the last milestone of an illness had been reached. This popular concept, with its accompanying anxiety, still permeates the thinking of the community and, consequently, of the individual patient who is part of that community. Furthermore, for the patient, hospitalization symbolizes an affirmation of his inability to deal with the demands of everyday living, an admission that his illness is not merely a temporary indisposition; and it may mean a confirmation of his fear that he is going to die. These fears are accentuated by separation from family and friends and by the need to abandon, at least temporarily, the normal pattern of living. As expressed by a well-known authority, "it is largely because the patient looks upon the hospital as a place where men groan and die, that the hospital is so often the clinical court of last resort." [1] The patient has to think of himself as part of a new world—the world of the sick.

What does it mean to be plunged suddenly into a world of illness? While the answer is as varied as the patients themselves, hospitalization carries with it certain implications to which all patients react. It is the way in which they react that varies from individual to individual.

The patient's first problems are related to the unfamiliar surroundings, the unaccustomed routines, the strange faces, the restrictions imposed by the hospital setting, and the fear of the unknown implicit in medical procedures. Later, as his stay lengthens, he becomes accustomed to his surroundings and begins to feel more at home. The strange world of the hospital becomes his world. As he becomes adjusted to living in this new world, the focus of his thinking shifts, and we find him preoccupied with other problems. Concern about the eventual outcome of his illness, his future employment, and his ability to support his family comes to the fore. He begins to wonder how long it will be before he can resume his accustomed place in the world and to doubt whether he will ever be the same again. The long separation from family and friends raises disturbing questions about the possibility of being forgotten by them, being dropped out of their lives,

[1] Bluestone, "Some Fundamental Problems in Hospital Administration," p. 515.

and losing the status which he may have attained with great effort.

Children are particularly vulnerable when faced with hospitalization. They too react to the unfamiliar surroundings with fear and bewilderment. For them, separation is even more threatening than it is for adults. Unable to understand the need for it, they view the parents' decision to leave them in the hospital as a sign of rejection and are filled with anxiety that they will be forgotten and abandoned.

STRANGENESS OF HOSPITAL LIFE

In order to understand fully the meaning of hospitalization for the patient, let us consider each one of these problems in greater detail. Let us look, first of all, at the need to adjust to life on a hospital ward.

When a patient enters a hospital, he enters a world totally different from the one to which he was accustomed and he has to learn to live in it, to become part of it. The large buildings, the long corridors, the sight of unfamiliar machinery, the white-clad doctors and nurses, the presence of so many other sick people, all are unfamiliar, bewildering, and all are frightening. To add to this strange, unfamiliar, and frightening feeling, the patient finds that he is no longer master of his own destiny; he has to give up personal control over even the simplest everyday functions. The time to get up, the time to go to sleep, what he will eat and when, with whom he will associate, whether the windows will be open or closed—these and other minutiae of everyday living are no longer determined altogether by his own likes and dislikes or habits built up in the course of a lifetime. Instead, they are now determined by an outside authority and have to be submitted to without question and without regard for personal preferences. He has neighbors to consider whose condition may be worse or better than his.

LACK OF UNDERSTANDING OF HOSPITAL PROCEDURES

The patient is subjected to examinations and tests, the purpose of which he does not understand and the results of which are not explained. A nurse comes in and sticks him with a needle, another one puts a thermometer in his mouth; a strange-looking machine is wheeled to his bedside and connected with his arms and legs; he is put on a stretcher and wheeled through long corridors and passageways. Some of the tests to which he is subjected are unfamiliar, some are painful, many are frightening, but nobody tells him what they mean. And nobody tells him whether the results are favorable or unfavorable. The patient is afraid to ask questions because everyone seems so busy, so intent on what he is doing. Or, perhaps he is afraid to ask because he is afraid to know the answer. Whatever the reasons, the unasked questions remain unanswered, and uncertainty and fear continue to prey on his mind.

Children as well as adults view the necessary medical procedures, which they do not understand and which are not explained to them, with apprehension. Though they are often unable to express their fears, they are afraid of pain and death. They may react with what appears to be inappropriate behavior because they misinterpret what they hear about their condition.

There was 10-year-old Johnny, for instance. A quiet cooperative boy, he submitted without protest to all the necessary procedures. Suddenly his behavior changed. He continued to be quiet and cheerful while in bed, but appeared to be filled with anxiety and terror whenever it was necessary for him to sit up. Frequently, he fought any attempt to make him do so.

It took a number of quiet talks with the social worker before he was able to discuss the reason for his fear. As Johnny explained it, he knew, for he had heard it said, that he had a leak in his heart—the doctor had mentioned a leaking valve. He was fearful that when he sat up, blood would drip through the hole, and when the last drop of blood leaked out, he would be dead.

Even the hospital practice of medical rounds, necessary as it may be for the training of medical staff and helpful in assuring thoughtful consideration of his medical problem, is not without its threats to the patient. It is true that the patient may feel that he is getting expert medical attention from the many physicians at his bedside and from the presence of the chief. Nevertheless, the discussion which ensues, and from which he is often excluded, the use of terminology which he does not understand, tend to arouse apprehension. He cannot help but speculate what it all means or what decision has been reached. Frequently, before he has had a chance to formulate the questions which come to his mind, the doctors have moved on to the next patient, if indeed they stopped at his bedside at all. They seem forever eager to see interesting and dramatic cases.

We have become more keenly aware of the effect the routine of hospital procedures has on the patient. Some years ago a forum on this subject was organized by the New York State Nurses Association. A newspaper article [2] in reporting the event describes the reaction of a "typical" patient on the panel as follows: "Patients would like to be thought of as people and not cases. Patients are already afraid when they enter hospitals and failure to explain routine and treat the sick person as an individual merely add to their fears. No one tells the patient 'who's who, or what's what,' " adding that a simple explanation of the necessity for many hospital procedures, if given to the patient when he enters the hospital, would immeasurably help his morale.

It was encouraging to find that the physician on the forum was in complete agreement with the "typical" patient's appraisal of the hospital situation. Doctors, nurses, hospital administrators, and other personnel, he said, work as a team

[2] New York *Herald Tribune*, March 31, 1950, p. 23.

and know what is going on. "But what about the patient?" he asked:

He is isolated from his world, from the people who take care of his emotional needs—his boss—his work—his wife—his business associates—his friends—the people who daily build him up, whether he be rich or poor. When he enters a hospital, his world is left pretty much outside. His needs must be met by the kindness, the sympathy and the understanding of those inside the hospital.

As one hospital administrator expressed it: "The fact which the average hospital employee does not grasp sufficiently is that he is judged by the sick man in accordance with his humanitarian rather than his scientific impulses." [3]

Such a point of view represents a newly awakened concern for the patient as a human being who, though ill, has needs in addition to the need for medical treatment. This concern is part of the increased appreciation of the effect of the patient's emotional state on his physical well-being and the obligation such an appreciation imposes for a more careful evaluation of what the prescribed and controlled hospital routine means to him.

ATTENTION TO THE NEEDS OF CHILDREN

The general concern with the patient's reaction to hospitalization and the need for help in this area is particularly evident in the changing attitude in dealing with hospitalized children. As more and more is known about the reactions of children, efforts are being made to remedy or eliminate the conditions which precipitate fear and misgivings. The personnel who work with youngsters are discovering various ways of helping to bring about a more satisfactory adjustment.

It was found, for instance, that a cheerful, nonhospital, nonthreatening atmosphere in the children's ward can dispel

[3] Bluestone, *op. cit.*, p. 517.

some of the child's anxiety. As a result, more and more frequently children's wards are decorated in bright colors with cheerful pictures painted on the walls. Most important, however, is the need to provide an extra measure of attention to allay the child's fear that he is unloved, unwanted, or abandoned. It has been found that while some children are so badly deprived emotionally that they turn to everyone around them for love and approval, most children respond best if there is one person to whom they can relate easily and to whom they can turn for reassurance.

Many new ways are being tried to satisfy the emotional needs of sick children, particularly if they have to remain in the hospital for long periods. Thus, in some communities, older people are being recruited to spend time with hospitalized children and act as "foster grandparents." While originally the program was organized to offer older people a satisfying activity and a means of earning extra money, it was found to be of great benefit to the children, particularly to those who were isolated, had few visitors, were immobilized, or presented feeding difficulties.[4]

The most effective means of alleviating children's anxiety lies in adopting preventive measures. In one community, for instance, groups of children are encouraged to visit the hospital for conducted tours. They are allowed to see many parts of the hospital and its facilities, to climb on the beds and to listen to a heartbeat through the stethoscope. Given such an introduction to the hospital, with emphasis on the fact that hospitals are places where people go to feel better, many children who must enter the hospital at a future date exhibit less anxiety than might otherwise be normal since the surroundings are familiar to them.

Equally important is work with the parents, both in understanding their own feelings about having a child hospitalized and helping them to prepare the child for the

[4] Davis, "Employing the Aged as Foster Grandparents in a Medical Setting."

experience. Individual contacts are made, group discussions are held, and pamphlets specifically designed for this purpose are distributed. Whatever means are adopted, the emphasis is on making a realistic preparation for the coming hospitalization and the necessary procedures.

A more difficult problem confronts the hospital personnel in dealing with the parent's personal problems in relation to the child and his illness. Such problems may center on manifest rejection of the child, as was the case with Mr. White. When he brought the child to the hospital for repair of a physical deformity it became easily apparent that Mr. White did not want the child, whom he blamed for his wife's death during childbirth. Such deep-seated rejection, whether openly expressed or concealed, requires prolonged treatment if there is to be a change of attitude.

Simple measures can help to overcome the parent's own anxiety about his child's medical condition, about the separation, or the type of care the child will receive. For instance, restrictions governing visiting hours are often removed, and the parent is encouraged to visit frequently In many hospitals arrangements are made to have the parent stay overnight with the child. This is particularly important during the early period of hospitalization. As the parent is reassured about the kind of care the child is receiving, and as the child is convinced that he is not being abandoned and that the parent will visit, the latter can return home, visiting only during the day.

ENFORCED DEPENDENCE

Those of us who work in hospitals have had ample opportunity to observe the effect of hospitalization upon the patient. The need to give up the right to make decisions both as to the details of everyday living and as to what is to be done to him, the physical demands of the illness, the feeling of helplessness, and the necessity to rely upon others for the satisfaction both of physical and of emotional requirements, all tend to center the patient's attention upon himself and to make him a completely dependent individual.

Traditionally, our society has emphasized the need to acquire independence as a prerequisite for growing up. We usually expect and assume that mature individuals have achieved a certain amount of self-sufficiency, have learned to take responsibility for their actions, and can decide what they consider best for themselves. The hospital patient finds that he is expected to relinquish suddenly and completely this self-sufficiency and independence which have been built up with difficulty, and over many years, as desirable social characteristics. In actuality, we are saying to him: "Disregard what you have been striving for all your life. In this situation you are no longer an adult, you become a child once again. You will be told what to do and when to do it, you will be cared for— you need only to submit."

How deep the regression to which hospitalization forces a patient is aptly described by Dr. Henry B. Richardson:

Entering a hospital does two things; the patient goes into a protective environment and he leaves the responsibility and stimulation of the home. . . . he is free from responsibility and also from less tangible things; the stimulation of books, of letters to write, the broken latch on the door requiring repair—everything indicating some potential activity. At the hospital his clothes are in a bag, his pajamas belong to the hospital, food is brought to him regularly, and the only thing he has to do is to carry out orders and this with an entirely passive attitude. If sick enough, he is brought a bedpan to attend to excretory functions . . . it is a startling comment on the hospital environment that going to a toilet is regarded as a "privilege." The patient does not start from scratch, but from the environmental age of a young child in terms of responsibility.[5]

If we assume that part of total medical care is to help the patient toward a more mature, more responsible attitude, it is important to remember than an adult is not a child and

[5] Richardson, discussion of "Psychosomatic Factors in Convalescence," p. 144.

should not be treated as one, even though illness may have forced him to give up some of the prerogatives associated with maturity. Nor should we expect him to maintain consistently a level of behavior which is usually associated with a mature individual. Illness, and particularly prolonged illness, may make it impossible for him to do so. Instead we must at all times accept and respect the level on which the patient himself can function and help him, in so far as possible, to reach the maximum of which he is capable.

Prolonged illness and hospitalization accentuate the regression characteristic of all illness. Separation from family and customary life experiences tend to withdraw the patient's interest from the world outside and to center it upon the illness and its manifestations. The longer the hospitalization, the more concentrated the attention on self and the greater the demands for similar concern from those around him. At the same time, the conduct of a busy hospital demands compliance with regulations for the protection of the group. Under pressure of these realistic requirements, we are likely to lose sight of the effect of such enforced dependence on the patient.

As we watch the patients, we see that their reactions differ. What is at the source of these reactions? What emotional needs are satisfied by the attention the patient is getting? What emotional needs are thwarted by the requirements of strict adherence to regulations and hospital routine? If we are to get answers to these questions, it is important to remember that the patient brings to his illness the same pattern of behavior and the same reactions that characterized him when he was well, even though the illness may bring these more forcibly to the fore. Such deep-seated emotional needs, and the patient's striving to meet them, cannot be eliminated merely by ignoring them. Nor can a satisfactory solution be found if we minimize their importance on the basis that we are dealing with a sick individual whose reactions are of little concern. It is only as we learn to understand the reasons underlying the patient's adherence to regulations, or defiance of them, that we can help discover more acceptable ways of adjusting him to the setting in which he finds himself. Certain medical procedures, unpleasant as they may be, are essential if adequate care is to be provided. Since they have to be undertaken at a time when in his struggle for life the patient is self-centered, it is important that they be done with his cooperation. Given such an understanding, and an awareness of the roots of the patient's attitudes and conflicts, his reaction to his illness, his need to accept or reject its reality, his fears and anxieties, we can help him toward the next step in emotional as well as physical recovery. Lack of such insight on the part of those entrusted with his care may well affect the patient's emotional state, and consequently his ability to profit by the medical treatment which will determine the very course of the illness and the eventual prognosis. The teachings of psychosomatic medicine must be borne in mind at all times.

If our theoretical knowledge of the roots of human behavior is to benefit the patient, and help him avail himself of the medical care at his disposal, it must be applied to the needs of the individual by translating it into action. In order to do this effectively, it is necessary to understand how the patient's inner needs are manifested in his acceptance or rejection of the adjustment the hospital requires of him.

Let us consider the "good" patient, the patient who submits without question, no matter how unpleasant or painful the experience may be. What is there in his life situation that accounts for his submissiveness? Is he an immature individual who has been denied the satisfaction of indulging his dependency and who now welcomes the dependent role assigned to him by his new experience? Do the illness and the protection of the hospital provide a welcome relief from a difficult social situation? Does the routine of hospital living, the extensive medical and nursing care, feed his need for love and affection by making him the center and focus of all attention?

What should be our approach to such a patient? Granted that a certain amount of dependency is necessitated by his physical condition, it is important not to forget that immaturity cannot be confined to one area alone. If we encourage regression to childhood and immaturity because it is convenient to have an obedient, cooperative patient for the smooth running of a hospital, we must then be prepared for a total regression to the same childish level. We must recognize that the patient, having accepted the dependency we foster, may at the same time become demanding of attention, complaining, disgruntled, and self-centered without the feeling of guilt which would otherwise accompany such behavior in a normal adult. If we understand that the "good" patient who does not give any trouble has regressed to a childishness which we have encouraged, we may then be able to accept without irritation his complaints or demands for attention as part of the same childish pattern.

On the other hand, we may have an independent, self-reliant patient who has long ago given up the pattern of childish dependency, who finds the restrictions irksome, and who rebels against them within the limits of his physical capacity. Does his resistance to the medical regimen have its roots in the same distrust and fear with which he might have met each new experience in the past? Do the restrictions, to him, mean merely an imposition of an outside authority and does he react to them as he has reacted to authority all his life? Or, is the patient fighting the restrictions imposed by his physical condition because by so doing he is rejecting the concept of himself as a sick person? Or does his resistance to the prescribed regimen have its roots in an unconscious desire to cling to his sickness? Is his presence in a hospital the best way for him to escape from an intolerable situation? And is he unable to abide by the restrictions because of his deep-lying, unconscious fear of getting well since this will, inevitably, bring him face to face with the same difficult situation he had escaped through his illness? Does his need to be sick spring from a desire to punish someone in his environment who hurt him, who does not appreciate him? Is he reacting like a child who strikes the chair against which he hurt himself? An understanding of the roots from which his rebellion springs will point to the way in which we can help him accept at least a measure of the dependency so essential for effective medical care, instead of merely insisting that he do as he is told "for his own good."

And what about the individual who has achieved the independence of maturity at great cost and after a long struggle? The precarious balance such an individual has managed to maintain can be seriously threatened by an imposition of restrictions which may precipitate an inner turmoil and rebellion reactivating the conflict between dependence and independence characteristic of the adolescent. The chain of reactions which this may bring in its wake is likely to influence the way in which he will use his illness and hospitalization. Since he has achieved but a semblance of maturity, the helplessness and dependence created by the illness might well play into his need to relinqish all responsibility and allow others to care for him.

There was Mr. F., for instance. He was a "good" patient, did exactly as he was told and made few demands. Despite extreme physical discomfort, he seldom complained. He explained that he did not want to complain, "because everyone was so good to him." He tried to ingratiate himself, and it was quite evident that he was constantly looking for approbation. Even though his illness threatened to leave him with a permanent handicap, he evidenced little concern about his future. Should he be unable to work, he said, he was sure someone would look after him—"there are good people in this world." The relief agency which took care of him while he was sick at home, just prior to hospitalization, would continue to care for him, he asserted glibly.

As we became better acquainted with Mr. F., we learned many facts about his past life which threw light upon his attitude toward his illness and the incapacity it produced. This was but a repetition of his previous pattern of dependency: first upon his mother, way beyond the age when such dependency is normal; later, upon his sister; and, more recently, upon his wife. The illness and stay in the hospital gave him an excellent opportunity to sink further into a dependency from which he was never adequately weaned. It was evident that he was ready to accept dependence upon the doctor, the social worker, and the relief agency as a way of meeting life's problems.

If the aim of total medical care is to accomplish more than to arrest the disease process, if it is to be really a means of rehabilitating this patient, a way will have to be found to wean him from a dependence which has been so satisfying in the past, and give him an incentive to wish to assume more self-responsibilty and more self-direction.

EFFECT ON CHILDREN'S DEVELOPMENT

It would appear at first glance that the dependence imposed by prolonged hospitalization is fraught with less danger for the child than for the adult, since the child is expected to be dependent. In reality, however, even for the child such prolonged dependence can create problems. In the course of his normal growth, the child is expected to assume gradually increased independence and more mature responsibility. Prolonged dependence imposed by illness can seriously interfere with this process of growing up.

The threat to the child's emotional and intellectual progress is being increasingly recognized, and means are being employed to provide the stimulation the child needs at different stages of his development. For instance, at the Convalescent Hospital in Cincinnati, toys and games are employed to help the child develop despite the constricted world in which he lives and to bring him in closer touch with the real world beyond the hospital walls. Appropriate toys are utilized to encourage creative ability, imagination in small children, and help them acquire new mental and manual skills, as well as to provide an outlet for display of emotion and release of feelings. Carefully selected games teach older children how to meet a challenge, and help to promote companionship with their peers.[6]

In another hospital, the Blythedale Children's Hospital in Valhalla, New York, where handicapped children remain for prolonged periods, an attempt is made to make the institution a "house on wheels." Here children continue their education in regular classes, from kindergarten through high school, attending in wheel chairs and movable beds which they learn to propel. In their free time they participate in a variety of games and activities. To create a normal atmosphere, children wear their own rather than hospital clothing. Parents are encouraged to visit often and to insure for the hospitalized child as much participation as possible in the normal life of the family, of which he is an important, though physically removed member.

Other institutions have similar programs, all of them designed to encourage the child with a prolonged illness or disability to develop to his fullest capacity.

FEAR OF TREATMENT PROCEDURES

The conflict between dependence and independence is not the only one the patient has to face. Other emotional components, present in all hospitalizations but particularly aggravated in the case of prolonged illness, are fear of the illness, of medical procedures, of possible death, and a sense of hopelessness. Even the patient who has accepted the need for hospitalization and for help with his medical needs is, as a

* Weyhmuller, pp. 68–70.

rule, not familiar with the specific procedures through which such help will be given. Each new procedure is, consequently, a threat because of the unknown it represents. The patient not only fears the pain and discomfort which may be involved but even more he fears what the procedure is likely to reveal.

There is little question but that these reactions may create trouble for the orderly conduct of the hospital and the rendering of effective medical care. Our concern for the welfare of the patient, however, will help us overcome such difficulties as the situation may present by constantly reminding us that troublesome as it may be for us, it creates even greater hardships for him. Here, as in so many other instances, the patient's reactions can be better understood and more easily accepted if we keep in mind that they are a part of his total personality as well as his way of meeting untoward situations.

There are definite steps which can be taken to minimize some of these problems. One of these is to give the patient, whether adult or child, not only an understanding of the meaning of the various procedures, but also a measure of participation in them and a sense of responsibility for carrying them out. He must be made to feel that he is not totally helpless. Given such an understanding of, and participation in, medical treatment, the patient's feeling of utter dependency, uselessness, and helplessness and the rebellion they create, can often be modified or even eliminated.

It is natural that when a person is sick, the opinion and support of the physician assume major importance for him. His entire mode of living is regulated by the doctor's recommendations. His present sense of well-being and his very outlook for the future are entirely dependent upon the doctor. As one patient expressed it, "My life is in their hands." The fact that the doctor in a busy hospital seldom takes the time to explain to the patient either the reason for, or the results of, the medical procedures tends to aggravate the patient's uncertainty and fear. The effect of this lack of sharing and the help which a social worker can give in such a situation are illustrated in the case of Mr. S.:

Mr. S. was referred to the social worker by the charge nurse who found him visibly upset following ward rounds. A discussion with the doctor revealed that Mr. S. had been depressed and withdrawn since his admission. The doctor questioned how much of this depression was part of the patient's usual personality pattern and how much of it might be a reaction to his illness and hospitalization. He asked for a detailed study of the patient's life as a help in understanding his attitude.

In talking with the social worker, Mr. S. expressed freely his disappointment at his failure to respond to treatment. What concerned him even more was the feeling that illness robbed him of his status. He was a professional man himself and felt that he would like to know "what it is all about." The doctor, he said, treated him as if his previous achievements were of no moment; as if his illness robbed him of his ability to understand and his right to make decisions. All the doctor saw was his illness; he was a "case," not a human being.

The patient's feelings were discussed with the doctor. Armed with this new understanding, the doctor made a conscious effort to discuss his findings and recommendations with the patient more freely. The patient responded eagerly. He became interested in the medical problem in an almost objective way and began to cooperate actively in treatment.

FEAR OF SURGERY

Frightening as are the unknowns of medical procedures, the prospect of surgery is even more frightening. Few people look forward even to minor operations without some misgiving. Patients with prolonged illness, already burdened by physical discomfort of long duration, often react to the recommendation for surgical intervention with apprehension and anxiety. They fear surgery per se, the additional discomfort and pain it is likely to create, the possibility of not surviving the operation, and the possible disfigurement and mutilation. Even more threatening are the long-range implications and the influence of deformities on familial and social relationships and job opportunities. This is particularly true when an amputation is being considered. The loss of a part of the body is not only traumatic in itself but, in addition, creates a sense of uselessness, a fear of permanent incapacity, and a feeling of difference.

Unfortunately, as in so many other instances, the patient is frequently excluded from any participation in arriving at a decision which vitally concerns him and may affect his entire life. Only too often, the doctor, having reached a decision, merely informs the patient that surgery is the only suitable method of treatment. All that is left for the patient to do is to sign a consent form. This approach merely serves to emphasize further his feeling of helplessness against overwhelming odds.

The decision as to whether to submit to surgery is often a difficult one for the patient to make. He is afraid to have the operation and he is equally afraid to risk the consequences of not having it. While the final decision has to remain with the patient, he can be helped to resolve his conflict and come to a decision if he is free to articulate his fears, to receive whatever reassurance is realistically feasible, and to weigh, as objectively as he can, the advantages and disadvantages. Even when the patient consents to surgery after a thoughtful weighing of the pros and cons, this does not obviate the possibility of a depression, nor the questioning in his mind about his ability to continue a meaningful and satisfying existence following it.

Once we understand the meaning an operation has for the particular patient with whom we are dealing, ways and means can be devised to demonstrate to him that his usefulness has not come to an end because of the loss of one particular part of his body and that he retains potentialities for useful living in spite of the handicap.

There was, for instance, Mr. I., a carpenter who felt that with a double leg amputation, his productive life had come to an end. He would never be able to work again, he was sure. He and his family would become objects of "charity."

Utilizing the services available in the hospital and as a preparation for Mr. I.'s return to the community, he was referred to the occupational therapy department. In planning for Mr. I. his former experience in carpentry was taken into consideration, and he was given toys to make. His dexterity was immediately apparent, and he derived considerable satisfaction from making toys for his children. This had meaning for him first and foremost because it showed him that his handicap was not the only thing that remained to him, that he was still able to use himself constructively. Furthermore, for some time past he had been deprived of his ability to provide for his family, and this was the first time in many months that he was able to give his children small gifts.

Every effort was made to utilize this successful experience as a demonstration of how useful he could still be. With encouragement, he regained some of his self-confidence and began looking forward to the time when he would be able, with the aid of a specially constructed bench, to use his newly acquired skill to earn a living and resume his old place in the family group.

FEELING OF EXCLUSION

Prolonged illness, necessitating, as it often does, prolonged hospitalization, poses a problem of separation from family and friends, totally different from what is encountered in acute illness. An acute illness with its dramatic onset and sudden removal to a hospital makes the patient the focus of attention and concern. For the overworked housewife, for instance, the secondary gains of an acute illness may be truly constructive, giving her an opportunity to be the center of attention and providing visible proof of the recognition implicit in her being missed at home. The concern of the family about her welfare may compensate her for the lack of recognition in her day-by-day job. By contrast, in prolonged illness, the patient may find that long before the illness is controlled, these secondary gains as evidenced by visits, gifts, and attention in general diminish and finally seem to vanish.

As these attentions decrease, hospitalization may begin to symbolize for the patient a desertion by his family. "To part is to die a little." And yet his needs are the same as those common to us all—the need to be useful, to be loved, to feel secure. Prolonged illness by its very nature is diametrically opposed to the satisfaction of these needs. The usual every-day satisfactions derived from normal family relationships, work experiences, and social contacts have to be given up for an indefinite period of time. Without their sustaining influence, the patient finds that the satisfaction of his inner needs is constantly interfered with. He feels frustrated and reacts to the frustration with tension and hostility.

The frustration caused by the temporary inability to earn a living, characteristic of any hospitalization, is aggravated when the illness is prolonged, for it carries with it the threat of permanent curtailment of working capacity. This inability to provide financially for his family, coupled with the expense imposed by long hospitalization, creates concern about the way they are managing. Some patients may be covered by workmen's compensation or private insurance. In both these instances, however, that compensation is minimal, and private insurance often excludes some of the prolonged illnesses. The recently enacted Medicare program relieves the patient of the greater part of the burden in meeting the cost of hospitalization. It does not, however, meet the needs of the family. Even reassurance that they are getting along is often not the entire answer, for it may mean a threat to the patient's adequacy and a fear that he is losing his rightful place in the family group.

As the illness progresses, especially if medical science is unable to arrest it or to ameliorate the distressing symptoms, the patient's fear that he may never be able to resume his place slowly develops into a certainty. This conviction is further enhanced by the family's tendency to exclude him by overprotection and by not sharing with him the vicissitudes of life, an exclusion to which the patient may react with hopelessness and despondency. As one patient put it, "They tell me nothing. It is as if I no longer exist."

Granted that in those instances where the chances of the patient's resuming his former place are slim, unrealistic reassurance is useless, even harmful. Nevertheless, complete exclusion, which fortifies his feeling of uselessness, is equally harmful. Those concerned with the patient's welfare must be helped to devise other means by which he can assert his worth as an individual and as a member of his family and of the community. Even when the patient's condition is such that improvement cannot be expected, every opportunity must be exploited to give him a feeling that he matters and that his debilitating illness and his confinement to a hospital bed in no way exclude him from participation in family living, nor affect his place in the family group. The following case is an illustration of the way in which such a situation was handled:

Mr. R. was in the hospital suffering from a progressive neurological condition.

The patient and his wife were an intelligent couple, apparently devoted to each other. When Mr. R. became ill, Mrs. R., an attractive, capable, and resourceful person, younger than her husband, secured a job easily and was able to maintain herself adequately. She was "lucky" to be able to work, she said, for she realized that the burden of support would fall upon her for an indefinite period. It was a relief to know that her husband did not have to worry about finances, that she was even able to show him little attentions, bring him gifts, make his stay more pleasant.

Despite this positive picture of a sustaining marital relationship and absence of financial worry, Mr. R. was invariably depressed and discouraged following his wife's visits. Given an opportunity to talk, Mr. R. had little difficulty in voicing his dejection to the social worker. As he put it, every time his wife visited him and tried to reassure him, it was borne more strongly upon him that he was "nothing but a stone around her neck." He had given her so little, for he became sick soon after their marriage. Now "she is tied to a helpless invalid."

Encouraged by the social worker, Mrs. R. too was able to voice her real feelings. She expressed freely her dissatisfaction with the situation in which she found herself. She felt all too keenly the burden of self-support, the need to work all day and take care of the home at the same time. While she would not want to miss visiting hours, she said, the long trip was exhausting and deprived her of any time for recreation. As she talked, she gave evidence of self-pity and a need for approval. Recognition for what she was doing was given unstintingly. It was acknowledged that she was carrying a heavy burden indeed.

Encouraged by the worker's understanding, Mrs. R. mentioned that in addition to her other troubles, her mother was sick and the doctor advised radiotherapy. She was worried and upset about her mother's illness, and did not quite know how to secure the necessary treatment since she could not afford to pay for it. She missed having her husband with whom to talk things over. She had always found him so helpful, and it was hard for her to do without his advice when she needed it. There was nothing to be done about it, she felt, since her husband was "too ill to be worried about other people's troubles."

Utilizing Mrs. R.'s concern for her husband's welfare, the social worker suggested that sharing her problem with him would not hurt him at all, but would make him see that he was not so useless as he imagined himself to be. He would derive satisfaction from knowing that he could help her. She was encouraged to draw him more into planning and to consult him whenever possible.

At first Mrs. R. was hesitant. She did not want to burden her husband with her problems. Gradually she began to realize that just because her husband was handicapped, it would mean a great deal to him to be of help to her. As her understanding of her husband's need grew, she not only began to discuss her problem with him and ask his advice but allowed him to take the leadership in planning.

PROBLEMS OF SPECIAL
DIAGNOSTIC GROUPS

The nature of the problems an illness poses for the patient is not related primarily to the diagnosis, but rather to the fact of the illness itself and the patient's reaction to it. Certain diagnostic groups, however, accentuate the severity of these problems for the patient. Among these problems are the fear of suffering and death, so prevalent among victims of cancer; the effect on family relationships and the fear of contagion, particularly marked in patients who have tuberculosis; and the feeling of hopelessness, seen so often in patients suffering from progressive degenerative diseases. A discussion of these diagnostic groups may prove helpful in focusing upon problems encountered in greater or lesser degree over and over again in every kind of illness.

FEAR OF SUFFERING AND DEATH

Cancer occupies a unique place among the "lingering" illnesses. To the community at large, a diagnosis of cancer was for a long time tantamount to a death sentence. It was the big "unmentionable," not to be referred to at all, if possible, and when this could not be avoided, to be mentioned in a hushed voice, a conspiratorial tone.

Times have changed to some degree. We find that the communication media show less reluctance to report that some known personality is suffering from cancer. More often, however, the fact is revealed after the death of the person involved. We know that medical knowledge has progressed to a degree to make possible successful treatment if the disease is discovered early enough. The fact, however, that the patient, following such successful treatment, has to return for periodic examinations to make sure that there is no evidence of the disease process cannot help but provoke anxiety for the patient himself as well as for those concerned with his welfare.

The fear of the disease therefore remains, as is evidenced by the fact that despite widespread publicity for the need of yearly examinations, not many take advantage of it, as if afraid to discover the "worst." As a result, many patients hospitalized with a diagnosis of cancer come to the attention of the medical profession at a time when succssful treatment may no longer be possible. Confronted with a feeling of helplessness at the present stage of our medical knowledge and the reality of unfavorable prognosis when the disease process is of long duration, the physician finds it difficult to discuss the diagnosis frankly with the patient.

It is true that there are other conditions where the prognosis is poor, but the doctor can say to the patient: "If you will take care of yourself, if you will do so and so, and avoid doing such and such, you have many years ahead of you." What can he say to the cancer patient who after months in the hospital is steadily and obviously getting worse? It is not surprising that often the doctor, frustrated by his own helplessness and unable to offer even the slimmest ray of hope, finds it difficult to talk about the diagnosis, and the patient's repeated question, "What is the matter with me?" is frequently met with evasion, a fact which settles nothing for the patient and merely serves to increase the already existing anxiety. While recognizing the difficulties this creates for the patient, it is important to remember that the doctor is not merely choosing the easier road for himself. Many physicians, because they fear the effect of such hopelessness on the patient's response to therapy, believe that it is unwise to divulge a diagnosis which, to most people, connotes suffering and imminent death. In addition, cognizant of the advances being made, they hope that some means of arresting the disease may be discovered in time to benefit the particular patient they are treating.

Whatever the doctor's thinking, he often believes that since the diagnosis has not been mentioned, the patient is not aware of it. And yet magazines and newspapers have made the community familiar with cancer symptoms, have discussed methods of treatment, and have emphasized that cures have been effected. The net result is that whether the doctor discusses it or not, many patients are aware of the diagnosis, many more suspect it.

Some patients cannot bring themselves to speak of cancer openly, but their awareness and anxiety manifest themselves indirectly. It is only as we learn to understand that a patient's discussion of cancer diagnosis in relation to other patients is but a manifestation of his knowledge and fear of his own condition, that his complaints about the hospital regimen, the treatment, the lack of attention, are but an expression of his discouragement, that we begin to see how much understanding he has of the nature of his own illness.

There are patients who mention openly that they have cancer. What concerns them and what they apparently want to talk about is their feeling of hopelessness, their fear of suffering and impending death. In the face of an anxiety which is realistically valid, false reassurance is not only futile, but negates what the patient knows to be true. Such negation carries with it a belittlement of the patient's suffering and of himself as a reasoning person. If the patient is to be helped, he needs an opportunity to voice his apprehensions, fears, and misgivings to someone who, accepting him as he sees himself, can remain sympathetic and yet not bcome emotionally involved.

This problem which is so prominent in cancer is not confined to this illness. It is evident in many other situations. There are indications that the medical profession is gradually changing its point of view about the value of the "medical lie," as indicated in an article in the New York *Times*. Under the title of "Medical Lie Opposed," the article quotes Dr. Walter C. Alvarez, retired senior consultant in the Division of Medicine of the Mayo Clinic, Rochester, Minnesota, as saying "that the patient is not deceived when assured that his critical illness left him in no danger." His own experiences in talking with dying persons, he said, convinced him that "they were so glad at last to have a friend with whom there was no need for keeping up the farce of constant makebelieve." [7]

The experience of social workers who have had occasion to work with cancer patients confirms this observation. Needless to say, this point of view does not impose upon anyone an obligation to be brutally frank at all costs and on all occasions. Rather it implies a willingness to listen to what the patient is trying to say, whether he actually articulates his fear or merely hints at it.

It would be natural to expect that the patient, when denied the opportunity to discuss his apprehension with his doctor, would turn to those closest to him—his family and friends. When he attempts to do so, he finds that under pressure of their own anxieties they may refuse to listen to his speaking of his fear of death. Their usual reaction is to try to escape the unpleasant situation by a complete denial of the possibility of such an outcome, by a reassurance which has no basis in reality, and an artificial cheerfulness which deceives no one and which fails to cheer.

It has been our experience that the opportunity to discuss his problems with someone who can bear to face the truth with him does more than reduce the patient's immediate fears and anxieties. It makes him feel less alone. What is even more important, having been given proof that the negative realities of his condition have been faced squarely with him, he can then accept, without questioning or misgiving, what-

[7] New York *Times*, March 21, 1951, p. 35.

ever reassurance can be given him as being equally valid. As an illustration, let us take the case of Miss J. and see how the social worker was able to help the patient without either affirming or denying the actual diagnosis:

Miss J., a cancer patient with metastasis to the bones, had been in the hospital for several weeks while tests were being made, medical work-up completed, and treatment instituted. A short while after treatment was begun, Miss J. spoke to the social worker about an article dealing with cancer which she read in a magazine. She readily identified the symptoms described as being similar to her own and drew the inference that she too was suffering from cancer. As she spoke about it, her anxiety and fear were clearly evident.

She had casually mentioned to the doctor, she said, that she thought she had arthritis. The doctor made her feel that she was probably right. And yet, he told her that the results of the tests had not yet come through. How could he know what the trouble was? Besides, she knew something about arthritis, and some of her symptoms did not "seem to fit in." Now she did not know what to believe or whom to trust. She suspected she had cancer; as a matter of fact, she was convinced of it. But how could she "really know" and be rid of the uncertainty once and for all?

No attempt was made either to affirm or deny Miss J.'s suspicion about her diagnosis. Instead, the worker tried to get from her a clearer understanding of what it meant to her. "If I have cancer, it means I am going to die soon. I am afraid of dying," she said.

It would have been easy at this point to tell Miss J. that she was wrong in her assumption; that the doctor had told her what he really thought; that she would soon be well again and that there was nothing to fear. Realizing that this would merely convince the patient that she was being deceived by everyone, the social worker concentrated not on the diagnosis, but on the feelings Miss J. expressed. Her fears and anxieties were accepted as real and understandable. It was pointed out, however, that if it were true that she had cancer at this time, she must have had it when she first came to the hospital and yet not only was she alive, she was responding to treatment. Every positive aspect of the patient's condition was utilized to show the progress she was making. The fact that she was now able to take care of her personal needs, wash, comb her hair, go for her treatments, whereas she had previously been bedridden, was stressed over and over again.

At the same time, the prolonged nature of her illness was mentioned. She was prepared for the fact that a smooth road to recovery could not be assured and that at times her condition might become worse. If this should happen, she could count on the hospital personnel to do everything possible to help her, as they had helped her in the past. Since regression was to be expected, this statement served to prepare Miss J. to meet any decline in her physical condition without the increased anxiety which usually accompanies such episodes.

Reassured by the worker's frankness and fortified by these concrete illustrations of every improvement evidenced so far, which she herself knew to be true, Miss J. was able to see that the diagnosis of cancer per se did not mean an immediate "death sentence," as she previously thought. After a while she was able to talk about cancer in the same way as another patient might talk about asthma, without the all-pervading fear which the diagnosis usually evokes.

FEELING OF HOPELESSNESS

Another group of patients who present serious problems are those suffering from progressive degenerative neurological conditions. These ailments frequently strike a young, economically productive group with families and young children dependent upon them. Unlike the prospects of some other patients with prolonged illness, such as cardiacs or diabetics, their prospects of returning to their traditional roles as providers are slim. For the most part they are aware of the progressive nature of their illness and slowly come to accept the fact that little can be done for them, their only remaining hope being in the possibility that some of the new experimental drugs may help.

Because of their feelings of hopelessness, utter inadequacy, and sometimes resignation, they present a variety of problems, particularly in the area of marital and familial relationships. Those patients who were family breadwinners prior to their illness have to face not merely a temporary inability to continue in that role but, in most instances, the realization that resumption of the previous role or even a modification of it is completely impossible. They are reduced to the status of helpless onlookers as they watch their families struggle on an insufficient public allowance, or see their wives trying to assume the burden of earning a living in addition to caring for the home and children. They frequently question how long a situation of that kind can last, how soon it will be before the wife, completely discouraged, will decide that the marital bond should be dissolved.

If he is not to give way to despondency, with concomitant repercussions on his medical condition, ways have to be found to demonstrate to the patient that despite his limitations he remains an individual who counts. As in so many other instances where the disease does not respond to therapy, where its progress is unrelenting and unrealistic reassurance impossible, it becomes necessary to draw upon and emphasize every positive aspect the situation presents. Getting the patient to help with family problems whenever possible, within limits imposed by the illness, is a concrete way to demonstrate his continuing usefulness and worth.

The story of Mr. G. demonstrates how helpful such an approach can be:

Mr. G.'s condition precluded any possibility of his ever assuming his old place in the family. Mrs. G. had made her adjustment. A capable, energetic person, she secured a job which enabled her to support the children, and had arranged her hours so as to be at home when the children came from school. The children were making satisfactory progress, and the father's absence from the home, at first a shattering experience, was no longer a factor in their lives.

Mrs. G.'s visits to the hospital were infrequent, the children's even more so. The family circle had closed, and Mr. G. was left outside it. Mr. G. often said that he could not blame his wife for not coming more frequently. "After all," he said, "she has her job, the care of the home and the children; she is tired, nobody could ask her to do more." He did not complain but he felt that his family "buried him before he was even dead." He appeared resigned to his fate.

That this resignation was only superficial, and that his need to carry some responsibility for the family continued, became apparent when he received word that Mrs. G. was ill. He was visibly upset because there was no one to care for her. And what would happen to the children? This was an opportunity to demonstrate to Mr. G. that despite his illness, he had a real contribution to make to those previously dependent upon him.

Since Mr. G. was ambulatory, special arrangements were made for him to go home on a pass several times within the month that followed. Now it was he who visited his wife and helped her a little while she was in bed, he who welcomed the children as they came home from school and reminded them to have their milk, he who arranged with a neighbor to come in and assist his wife.

When he returned to the hospital after the second visit, Mr. G. came in to see the social worker. For the first time the façade of hopeless resignation crumbled, and he broke down as he told the worker that at last he felt "like the man in the family once again."

In the case of female patients, the same medical problems often produce somewhat different reactions. Although obliged to give up their traditional role of mother and "doing for the family," they seem to be able to hold on to their role of ruling the family's destiny. Even from a hospital bed, they handle problems of household management with a spirit of possessiveness which belies their physical incapacity. Fortified by the cultural pattern of the woman being entitled to care and attention from the husband, we find them demanding, complaining, and forcing their husbands to show them attention as a means of preserving their status.

Tuberculosis, like cancer, was at one time an illness only to be whispered about. The campaign of public education has succeeded in eliminating, to some extent, the stigma previously attached to the illness, but much of this feeling still remains. In addition, the reality problems with which the disease confronts the patient and all those closely connected with him are numerous and impinge upon many areas. The magnitude and variety of the social problems that confront the tuberculous patients are so well recognized that tuberculosis has become known as a "social problem with medical aspects." The emotional aspects and physical manifestations of the illness are closely interwoven so that there is a never-ending cycle of interaction which may seriously affect the actual progress of the disease. According to eminent authorities in the field of psychosomatic medicine:

It has not been sufficiently stressed that there are emotional patterns which are related to eating habits, appetite and nutrition, and that these may be responsible for the underweight with which many cases of pulmonary tuberculosis begin. Furthermore, anxiety may prevent adequate sleep and rest. Finally, the shallow respiratory excursion seen in certain neuroses may play some role in this disease. These and probably other emotional factors should be considered in the etiology of pulmonary tuberculosis.[8]

In the majority of instances, tuberculosis strikes people in the productive years of life and interferes with their earning capacity not only in the immediate present, but for an indefinite period to come. Many of the patients are preoccupied with problems of adequate financial provision for the family, maintenance of the home, the care of children. These problems are of concern to patients in any prolonged illness, but until recently were aggravated even further for this particular diagnostic group. The period of hospitalization was usually longer than for many other ailments, and

[8] Weiss and English, p. 615.

most of the patients knew enough about tuberculosis to be fully aware of this fact. They were also aware that such lengthy hospitalization was unavoidable and that substitute arrangements were, for the most part, impractical.

Within recent years the widespread use of drugs, namely streptomycin, *p*-aminosalycylic acid and isoniazid has resulted in a considerable decrease in tuberculosis mortality, shortened the period of bed rest, and in many cases eliminated the need for prolonged hospitalization. However, these spectacular results are confined in the main to those cases where the damage is minimal and where the patients can be relied on to follow a strict regimen on an outpatient basis. Most of the problems with which the illness confronts the patients and their families, and which will be discussed in the pages that follow, still exist though their severity is minimized when drug therapy proves effective.

What are these problems?

Because the patients in the main fall into a young age group, and because of the contagious nature of the illness, the continuation of the marital relationship and their status as parents are frequently threatened. The contagious aspect of the illness creates numerous problems. A patient who has to avoid all physical contact, who is forbidden to express his affection in the usual way, whose dishes have to be sterilized, necessarily feels keenly his separation from normal social contacts, from family and friends. He feels cast out by his family and by society, unwanted, segregated, unclean. That the patient's concern is no idle fear is illustrated by what happened to Mr. N.:

Shortly after the diagnosis of tuberculosis was established, Mrs. N., fearful of the effect of her husband's illness on herself and their two small children, decided that she did not want the relationship continued and secured a legal separation. Mr. N. felt this rejection keenly. He was able to bear it only by blaming his wife for what he considered her refusal to carry her part of the burden and stressed particularly the fact that he had always been a good husband and provider.

How much it actually meant to him was also shown by the steps he took to keep his condition a secret from all those whose opinion he valued. He insisted that his children be told that he had gone away for further training in his trade as radio mechanic, for he was afraid that should they know of his condition, they might never want to have anything to do with him. His friends were told that he left for another city because of a better job opportunity. "I want neither their sympathy nor their loathing." In talking of his future plans, he mentioned that when he was discharged, he intended to go far away, to the West Coast maybe, "where no one knows me or my trouble." Feeling lonesome and deserted, he reached out to other patients but retreated as soon as there was evidence of a real friendship developing. As he put it, "I don't want to be hurt again."

This is not an isolated instance. While legal separation, representing as it does complete family disintegration, does not occur too often, a refusal on the part of the spouse to have the patient come home, on pass or when discharge from the hospital is recommended, is not unusual. Even though the fear of contagion is given as the reason, the patient detects the rejection underlying the refusal, and it increases his feeling of personal undesirability.

In the fight against the spread of the disease, both the medical profession and popular writers have put considerable emphasis on the need for the sick person to take elaborate precautions to protect others. This puts the burden of responsibility on the patient, adding to the heavy burden he is already carrying. The patient cannot help but be concerned lest, unwittingly, he might have been responsible for communicating the disease to others among family and friends, and he feels guilty as a result. On the other hand, if another member of the family had tuberculosis, the patient may develop an understandable resentment that lack of proper precautions brought about his own predicament.

NEED TO NEGATE ILLNESS

In many instances, a diagnosis of tuberculosis comes as a shock, and the patient is rushed off to a hospital before he has had an opportunity to absorb the new knowledge and its implications. Fear and anxiety are the usual concomitants of the illness, sometimes expressed directly, at other times covered up more or less successfully. The difficult initial adjustment to hospitalization is further complicated by the erroneous information that patients gather from the popular press about the nature of the illness, its stages, the significance of different symptoms, and the usual medical treatment. Having learned, for instance, that a positive sputum is a definite indication of tuberculosis, they find it difficult to accept the fact that even though their sputum is negative, it does not mean that they are well, nor that a single favorable x-ray examination is not, of itself, an indication of cure. Consequently, in the past they were bewildered and resentful when they were not allowed to leave the hospital as soon as the results of the x-ray examinations were negative.

As a result of these misconceptions and their anxieties about themselves, we find that patients exhibit an insatiable desire for information, are never quite satisfied with the explanations given them, and ask the same questions over and over again. Unless the patient's underlying anxiety is understood, his attitude may create serious friction with the physicians and other hospital personnel.

In tuberculosis a realistic acceptance of the illness is a prime essential if treatment is to be effective. The patient must not only allow medical procedures to be instituted, but must participate actively in carrying out the physician's recommendations. There are, however, patients who despite their knowledge of the diagnosis are unable to accept all that it implies. How this inability to accept the reality of the illness can influence treatment is illustrated in the case of Mrs. K.:

This patient was seen by the social worker on the day following her admission. From the medical chart the social worker knew that Mrs. K. had a diagnosis of bilateral tuberculosis—far advanced. In talking with the worker, however, Mrs. K. indicated that she either did not know or, more likely, was unable to accept the true nature of her illness. According to her statement, she had been sent to the hospital by her private physician "for observation" and would be returning home "within a few days." She appeared calm, collected, and cheerful.

The social worker recognized that in giving this distorted picture of her situation, Mrs. K. was in reality trying to negate her illness and all that it implied. By so doing, however, she was at the same time negating the need to help in the medical treatment so essential for her welfare. Recognizing the importance of the patient's participation, it became the social worker's responsibility to help this patient face the reality which confronted her. She knew, however, that merely forcing Mrs. K. to face a reality which was unacceptable to her would accomplish little beyond arousing negativism. It was only by slow stages, by discussing the "temporary" arrangements made for the care of the baby, that the patient's true concern was brought to the surface.

Behind the patient's controlled exterior lurked a fear that she did not dare admit even to herself—a fear that her illness was perhaps something serious, not merely a matter of "a few days." If that were the case, many other problems would clamor for solution. There was her young husband. What would it mean to him and to their future together? And what would happen to her 10-months-old baby? It was easier to push these thoughts away, not to have to deal with all these unpleasant and disturbing complications.

As Mrs. K., in discussing her problem over a period of time, became aware that there was someone to help her, she was better able to articulate her fears and misgivings. The overwhelming nature of the problem may have been too much for this patient to face alone and unaided, and so she had to negate it completely. Convinced that there was someone on whom she could count for help and guidance, she was able to accept what her illness implied and turn her energies to helping the doctor help her.

For those patients whose disease is advanced and does not respond to drug therapy, the very treatment, both the inactivity of bed rest and surgical procedures, major and minor, holds threats. Even when they apparently recognize the importance of bed rest, patients become impatient after a while because "nothing definite is being done." In their fear of what the illness may do to them, patients frequently react to enforced bed rest with hostility, for they feel that treatment which might be beneficial is being withheld. The way in which inner turmoil and tension can undo all the advantages of physical rest is so well known that it does not require any elaboration here. The patient who is advised by the doctor to "rest and not worry" may be able to follow directions so far as physical activity is concerned. However, a patient can hardly be expected not to "worry" when his mind is preoccupied with the economic insecurity of his family, with the fact that the marital partner has not been visiting frequently of late, when he is concerned that he is becoming a stranger to his children. This is particularly true when days and weeks pass and the patient does not feel any improvement and when nothing specific is being done for him. In the presence of such inner turmoil, how realistic can the "rest" be? Tensions and worries normally find release in physical activity. Deprived of the freedom to pace back and forth or to engage in any occupation to "take his mind off his troubles," the patient is restless and dissatisfied, twisting and turning in his bed. Thus all the advantages of the prescribed physical rest may be undone, for it has been demonstrated that the patient actually expends as much physical energy in such activity as he would have if he were up and about.

On the one hand, patients often resent the inactivity of bed rest; on the other, they become apprehensive and agitated whenever a new medical procedure is contemplated, fearing both the pain involved, as for instance in bronchoscopy, as well as the implications for the future. As in all other medical conditions, this apprehension is intensified when surgery is proposed. As in all surgery, the threat of the danger involved and the uncertainty of its success are aggravated by concern over cosmetic results—the effect the disfigurement might have on marital relationship, attitude of children, social contacts. The fact that the possibility of surgery is usually known by the patient long before the procedure is actually carried out serves to aggravate and intensify the anxiety, keeping him in a state of agitation and uncertainty.

LEAVING THE HOSPITAL AGAINST MEDICAL ADVICE

Prior to the advent of drug therapy, there existed a considerable problem in relation to the patients who discharged themselves prematurely against medical advice. For instance, a study sponsored by the New York Tuberculosis and Health Association in 1947 [9] revealed that over one third of these patients left against medical advice.

The reasons for leaving were analyzed, and it was found that primary among them was the patient's concern about his family relationships. This concern may take two forms. On the one hand, there is the patient who is worried about the family's economic security and his inability to provide financially. On the other hand, there is the patient who is disturbed by the very fact that the family is managing without him and fears the loss of security and standing it implies for him. The longer the separation, the more acute the feeling of

[9] Drolet and Porter, p. 9.

loss of status and security. The patient who is the victim of such insecurity and who is prompted by his need for reassurance may insist upon returning home before he is medically ready to do so, as if to test his family's love and their willingness to have him back.

In commenting on these findings, the statement was made that:

The treatment of tuberculosis requires long periods of restricted physical activity and enforced rest. During this time mental and emotional energies remain as active as ever, especially in individuals still in the prime of life. One way in which many patients reacted to this situation was found in their extreme concern over their husband or wife, children or other members of the household. The longer the hospitalization period, the more likely are changes in the family situation to occur; and whatever these may be, the greater the concern and the patient's desire to return home.[10]

Since it is important to help the patient to remain in the hospital, if his condition is to be treated, an attempt has to be made to remove the pressure of some of these familial situations and provide an opportunity for continued medical treatment, as illustrated by the case of Mr. W.:

At the age of 29, Mr. W. found himself in the hospital suffering with tuberculosis. The implications of the diagnosis, the need for prolonged and absolute rest, were not unknown to him, for his wife had been released from a tuberculosis sanatorium but a short time before he himself became ill.

Not only was Mr. W., a skilled worker, the provider in the family, but his wife's illness of several years' duration imposed upon him the role of the strong person on whom his wife could lean. It was he who took care of her when she first became sick, who made plans for the care of the child, who visited her in the hospital, and who watched over her when she returned home. His illness suddenly confronted him with a reversal of roles. It was one thing to accept dependence in his wife; that situation

[10] *Ibid.,* p. 42.

even gave him a certain amount of satisfaction, for it fitted in with his need to be the strong person. It was quite another matter to accept such a dependence for himself and to watch Mrs. W. assume the major responsibility, have her visit him in the hospital and bring him gifts, make all the decisions, and try to protect him from all unpleasantness.

As one observed Mr. W., he appeared to be an excellent patient. Eager to abide by the doctor's recommendations, he talked rather glibly about his understanding that it would be necessary to remain in the hospital until the doctor said he was ready to resume the care of his family.

As time passed, Mr. W. began to show signs of restlessness. He discussed the prospect of leaving the hospital more and more frequently. He maintained that his wife was lonesome, she needed "cheering up," she could not manage her everyday affairs without his help. A day came when, unable to cope with his inner turmoil, Mr. W. announced that, regardless of the doctor's advice, he was going to leave the hospital.

Such an action on his part was in direct conflict with the demands of his physical condition, the complete inactivity, the relaxation and further medical treatment it required.

Had the social worker been conscious of these physical aspects alone, she would have emphasized the need for complete rest, relinquishment of responsibility, and concentration on medical treatment. Such advice often given to patients by well-meaning friends and relatives has proved its ineffectiveness in the past, for it ignores the effect of emotional tensions on physical well-being.

To be of real help to this patient, the social worker had to discover what satisfactions could compensate Mr. W. for the loss of his usual satisfactions. What could be done to alleviate his feeling of being excluded and help him maintain his self-respect and consciousness of status as an individual and head of his family, so important to him?

Instead of advising Mr. W. "not to worry" about his family, advice he obviously could not follow, the social worker recognized Mr. W.'s concern as legitimate and valid. Even though she was unable to restore Mr. W.'s status as provider, she succeeded in giving him recognition as head of the family by consulting him in all matters pertaining to their welfare, seeking his participation in planning for them, and helping him to help Mrs. W. adjust to his absence.

Relieved of the anxiety created by what he considered to be his loss of status, Mr. W. was slowly helped to build up new values for himself and to see that ability to provide was not the only criterion by which to measure his value to his family. In view of the prolonged nature of his illness such a substitution was important not only during the period of hospitalization, but also for his future well-being.

Closely allied with his feeling about status as head of the family was Mr. W.'s feeling about his job and the success he had attained in it. The worker utilized the fact that the employer was holding the job open for him to reinforce Mr. W.'s opinion of himself as an adequate, valuable worker. Similarly, his fellow employees' interest in Mr. W., as exemplified by their many attentions to him, was used to emphasize his position of importance and value as a member of the larger community group.

The importance of preserving whatever satisfactions Mr. W. could derive in spite of his illness during his period in the hospital is self-evident. More important, however, is the effect these satisfactions had on Mr. W.'s ability to take advantage of the medical treatment. He was able to accept more easily the dependence imposed by his illness as he slowly acquired the conviction that in spite of it, his status in the family was being maintained. Under these circumstances, it was no longer necessary for him to fight the medical recommendation for prolonged rest; for he had learned that even when confined to a hospital bed he could continue to be a real force in his family's life.

Studies indicate that concern about family relationships was not the only factor responsible for the practice of leaving the hospital against medical advice. Listed among the other factors was the patient's dissatisfaction with the medical procedures, the attention received, the entire hospital routine, and his unwillingness to follow medical advice regardless of his reasons for it. Whatever the source of these dissatisfactions, we must recognize that little can be accomplished merely by insisting that the patient comply with what is recommended for him. The worker in the field of medical care is the last person in the world to behave like a martinet. The discipline of the sick is different from the discipline of the well. When the resistance to medical orders and the resulting dissatisfactions stem from a long-standing negative reaction to authority, as is so often the case, it can be readily seen that countering the patient's complaints with a further reenforcement of authority will merely serve to fortify his decision to do as he wishes.

Whether it stems from concern over family affairs or discouragement in the face of lack of improvement, if the severity of the problem of discontinuing medical care prematurely is to be reduced, and patient and community protected, it is essential that we have an awareness of the factors contributing to the patient's decision to leave the hospital before treatment is completed.

It is not enough to attempt to "educate" the patient. Nor can we assume that because we are dealing with an intelligent individual he will be able to make a "sensible" decision. In many instances, the patient is undoubtedly fully aware of all the good and logical reasons we can advance. Such an intellectual approach is often fruitless because it fails to get at the root of the problem. Something beside the patient's intellect is involved. It is only as we are able to understand the patient's feelings and help him in that area that any actual progress can be made. In this connection the report of the New York Tuberculosis and Health Association states: "Those dealing with tuberculous patients must keep in mind the interrelationship of physical, social and emotional factors of treatment and by so doing will be better able to contend with those problems arising from treatment." [11] With this as a background, the patient can be given help through an

[11] *Ibid.*, p. 50.

impartial presentation of the penalties involved, leaving to him the choice, if he is in a position to make a choice, of alternatives, and the right to make the ultimate decision. Given such a choice, relieved of the pressure of authority imposed from without, the patient's decision is more likely to be based on a real appraisal of what is involved rather than on blind impulse motivated by an unconscious resistance which obscures judgment. A promise that any reasonable complaint will be resolved promptly often accomplishes this purpose. To illustrate what can be done to help a patient follow the doctor's recommendation, let us consider Mr. A.:

A 35-year-old man with a wife and two children, Mr. A. was admitted to the hospital with minimal tuberculosis, responded well to bed rest, and was awaiting transfer to a sanatorium. His wife, though finding it difficult to manage on public assistance, tried to hide the truth from the patient, not wanting to upset him. However, the patient soon guessed the true state of affairs, "not so much from what she said, as from what she failed to say." There was only one thing for him to do, he decided, and that was to return home and take care of his family.

The danger inherent in such a procedure was pointed out to Mr. A. and the suggestion made that he and his wife talk over the situation and together arrive at some plan.

Mrs. A., a dependent person who always looked to the patient for advice and guidance, was able to accept the limitations imposed by her situation, once her husband's moral support was restored to her. The patient, reassured that with his help his wife would be able to carry on, and convinced that he could help most by submitting to treatment, abandoned his original intention to sign out against medical advice and remained in the hospital until treatment was completed.

Though no actual alteration in the situation was possible, the handling of the problem restored to the patient his status as head of the family while at the same time relieving the wife of the need to carry a heavy burden alone.

The shorter hospitalization made possible by drug therapy resulted in a reduction in the number of patients leaving the hospital against medical advice. In those instances, however, where the response is slow and the patient's need for prolonged hospitalization continues, this problem persists.

As one reviews the variety and complexity of the problems which prolonged illness imposes, one cannot escape the conviction that the lot of the hospitalized patient is indeed not a happy one, even in the best of circumstances. Granted that there are certain distinct advantages to being in the hospital, that certain treatment can be administered only in the hospital, and that certain restrictions are unavoidable, it is essential that we have a clear understanding of how the patient's emotional problems affect his response and influence his ability to make the best use of the medical facilities available for his care, prolong the process of recovery, and exact a heavy toll from patients and family members alike. Such an understanding can be arrived at only through an appreciation of the interrelation of the patient's social, emotional, and medical needs. An effort to mitigate in so far as possible the harmful effects of the problems created by hospitalization becomes the responsibility of the professional team concerned with the patient's care, working hand in hand with those most closely concerned with the patient—his family.

6

POSTHOSPITAL ADJUSTMENT

Hospitalization normally represents but a brief interlude in a person's life. Even assuming the best possible hospital adjustment with a minimum of the fears and anxieties we have been discussing, the hospitalized patient looks forward to his return home as a natural goal.

As in practically every other aspect of medical care, the situation is somewhat different for the patient with prolonged illness than it is for his acutely ill counterpart. In acute illness, once the episode which brought him to the hospital is over, the patient is usually ready to resume normal living following a short period of recuperation. Not so the patient with prolonged illness. The ongoing disease process means that at the end of his hospitalization, the patient is faced with a new set of problems. For him, discharge from the hospital does not, as a rule, imply recovery; for the very nature of the illness admittedly means, at best, a delayed "cure." Even though the acute episode has subsided and the progress of the illness has been temporarily arrested, the illness itself may continue as long as he lives and gradual deterioration or an acute flare-up can be expected. In other words, for the patient with prolonged illness, hospitalization is not an isolated, temporary experience to be forgotten once he leaves the hospital. Rather, it is but one of the stages in a life which henceforth will be governed by the demands of an illness which threatens to change the whole pattern of living.

TREND TOWARD
SHORTER HOSPITALIZATION

The very concept of "discharge" from a hospital for prolonged illness is of comparatively recent origin. In the past, the fact that the illness was chronic in nature and the prognosis poor influenced our over-all thinking about the patient and, consequently, the provisions made for his medical care. Even when such a patient entered a hospital for active medical treatment, he was likely to remain there indefinitely on a custodial basis, because of the prevailing easy-going medical attitude.

We are witnessing a shift in emphasis, restricting the use of hospital beds to those patients who are able to profit by active medical care. At the same time, there is a growing trend toward curtailment of the period of hospitalization in the treatment of prolonged illness for the same reasons that it has been shortened for the acutely ill patient. Several factors are responsible for this general trend toward shorter hospital stays and earlier discharges. Foremost among these factors are the developments which have been occuring in the science of medicine. New methods of treatment tend to facilitate earlier ambulation following even major surgical procedures. There is a growing conviction that continued hospitalization and bed rest, important as they may be at certain stages of the illness, reach a point of diminishing returns and, if prolonged unnecessarily, may even prove detrimental to the patient's welfare. At the same time, there is better recognition of early symptoms exhibited by the patient and a growing appreciation of the importance and effectiveness of early diagnosis and treatment. As a result, there is a greater tendency on the part of medical practitioners to hospitalize their patients before the illness goes out of control or becomes critical.

The popular concept of hospitalization has also undergone perceptible changes. The hospital is accepted more easily as the normal, indeed the desirable, place for people suffering from certain kinds of sickness. This acceptance has resulted in the referral of ever larger numbers of patients for hospitalization, straining facilities to the utmost. The consequent overcrowding and the ever mounting cost of hospital care thus make imperative a more productive utilization of available beds, necessitating a clearer differentiation between the patients who are in need of active medical treatment and those in need of custodial care.

In addition, members of the hospital staff, becoming increasingly aware of their need to know more about prolonged illness, tend to utilize the hospital experience as an opportunity for learning, and press for the removal of those patients who can no longer profit by active medical treatment. As a result, hospitals that minister to patients with prolonged illness are disassociating themselves more and more from the treatment of patients who require only custodial care, and are beginning to think of themselves as centers of treatment, teaching, and research.

THE PATIENT'S ATTITUDE TOWARD DISCHARGE

The community as a whole has failed to keep pace with this changing concept of medical care and continues to think of the patient suffering from a prolonged illness as requiring indefinite confinement within a hospital. The patient, naturally, mirrors the attitudes of the community of which he is a part and reacts with doubt, bewilderment, and questioning when confronted with the statement that there is nothing further the hospital can do, and with the recommendation that he leave the hospital. The patient's confusion is understandable if we bear in mind that frequently his condition may have been improved but slightly by the hospital stay, and the visible physical gains may be negligible. Nor can we disregard the effect produced by the realization that the doctor is unable to help him.

In view of the all-pervading influence of prolonged illness, it is not surprising to find that discharge from the hospital poses problems for the patient, as well as for all those closely associated with him. What the patient's reaction to this situation will be, what adjustment he will be able to make, will be determined in part by his actual physical condition and the amount of activity he is capable of undertaking, in part by what awaits him in the world outside, and in part by his emotional make-up and his usual way of meeting life experiences in general.

Patients vary in their ability to relinquish the dependence and attention which go with prolonged hospitalization. In the same way that the patient's emotional needs determine his acceptance or rejection of the hospital experience, so will they exercise their influence on the way in which he will face discharge and return to a more independent existence. An understanding of the patient's inner needs and the satisfactions he seeks from life is, therefore, a prime essential if we are to understand why one patient will deny the illness and what it means, see only the hopeful aspects, and be blind to all its implications, while another will exaggerate symptoms, cling to the illness and his infirmities, and stubbornly refuse to give up his invalidism.

For those patients who feel inadequate in the face of the competiton and trials of the workaday world, discharge may represent a threat; for it means that they are once again being brought face to face with the problems from which hospitalization removed them. No matter how unsatisfactory the hospital experience may have been, the world outside may be even more threatening. It is, therefore, not surprising that even those patients who have had difficulty in adjusting to the hospital may react with fear, anxiety, and resistance to the prospect of leaving its protection.

Prolonged hospitalization, with its need to comply with the regimentation of life in the hospital, separation from family and friends, the feeling of anonymity, helplessness, the constant presence of other sick people, imposes a heavy burden upon the patient. He is, however, able to derive some consolation from his conviction that this is but a temporary situation, if he can get himself to feel that way. No matter how bleak the situation is at times, he can hold on to the hope that once the hospital experience is over, he will resume his place in the world outside. Now, having come to the end of his hospital stay and recognizing that he is not cured despite months of care, the patient may reasonably question the decision that he is ready to return home when the goals he has hoped for have not been reached.

Some patients may view the decision that they are ready for discharge merely as an attempt on the part of the hospital to "get rid" of them. Unfortunately, all too often the attitude of the hospital personnel is such as to fortify the patient's feeling of being unwanted. Pressed by the need to serve the more acutely ill patients, and knowing that there is little more they can do for him, doctors and nurses tend to neglect the patient who is about ready to leave. Thus, the security of their interest and concern is removed at the very point at which the patient's anxieties are at their height. There exists a prevailing notion that every patient looks forward to leaving the hospital, and yet the reactivation of symptoms, so frequently seen when discharge is considered, is eloquent testimony to the patient's reaction to this withdrawal of interest and to the struggle within him:

A dramatic example of this type of reaction was provided by a 60-year-old woman who, following an uneventful postoperative recovery, was recommended for discharge. She advanced numerous arguments why she could not leave the hospital: she was still sick; she needed attention which she would not be able to get at home; and so on. Every attempt was made to change her attitude, every possible encouragement was tried, but no change could be effected. Finally, a definite date for discharge was set, but the day before she was to leave the patient fell out of her wheel chair and fractured an arm. The accident, however, did not seem to disturb her; her only comment was, "I cannot possibly go home now."

The reaction to discharge is not always so overtly or dramatically expressed. More often it manifests itself indirectly, either in difficult or placating behavior, or in open hostility toward the hospital for the "unjust" treatment, or sometimes even by the statement that "if this is the kind of hospital it is, I am glad to be through with it."

PROBLEMS THAT CONFRONT PATIENTS
AT DISCHARGE

No matter what the patient's initial reaction may be, it remains true that the adjustment he is called upon to make is a difficult one. If we are to help the patient give up the protection provided by the hospital experience without overwhelming fear, without embittering resentment, and with some semblance of hope and faith in the future, we need to offer him an acceptable goal, with some means of achieving a sense of security and of finding satisfactions in the world outside. Such satisfactions may be difficult to provide in view of the very real problems these patients have to face. Many of them seek answers to such questions as, "Where do I go from here?" and "Where can I get the medical care I still need?" It is not always possible to find satisfactory answers to either of these questions.

NEED FOR ADEQUATE LIVING ARRANGEMENTS

Those patients who have no families or who have severed their ties with relatives may have no place which they can call "home." Some of them lived alone prior to their illness in furnished rooms or small apartments. This arrangement, satisfactory as long as they were able to care for themselves, proves no longer feasible when outside help with everyday needs is an essential prerequisite to remaining in the community. Even the existence of family ties does not prevent difficulties from arising. Where the marital tie is not a strong one, the helplessness of the patient may serve as the precipitating factor in a complete family disintegration. Fear of the illness, concern about contagion, the fact that the marital partner may not be able to give the patient the attention he requires—all these may be real considerations or may be given as reasons to cover up the rejection of the patient and the family's unwillingness to have him return to the home.

The problem becomes particularly aggravated when the patient is elderly, or when the spouse is dead, or too old and too feeble to undertake the care of a seriously disabled mate. Even where there are adult children who have their own homes, difficulties might arise to prevent their making a home for an ailing parent. Whether the inability to provide a home is realistically valid or is based on unadmitted, sometimes even unconscious, unwillingness prompted by an underlying rejection, it creates problems which cannot be solved merely by exercising pressure on the family members. If the goal is to assure a satisfying life for the patient, leaving the hospital becomes but the first step. The patient must feel that he is not merely going away from the hospital, but that he is going where he will feel wanted, safe, and comfortable. It is only as the patient is made to feel that his relatives are willing to accept him and make a home for him that we can expect him to overcome the feeling of rejection implicit in the hospital discharge without too much anxiety and with some hope for what the future holds for him.

Even under the most favorable conditions, sharing the home of relatives may be a difficult experience for the patient. Accustomed to independent living, the patient finds that he must give up his independence and freedom and adjust his way of life to the needs and desires of others. Sensitive to the change from a self-sufficient, normally functioning individual to one who can no longer care for himself and constantly needs the help of others, the patient has the ever present consciousness of being a burden. Faced daily by his disability and inadequacy among those who knew him in his prime, to whom he represented a strength on which they could lean, the patient cannot help but question his ability to retain their love and respect. Not only does the patient have the normal need to be wanted, to be loved, and to be useful, regardless of his limitations, but this need may be accentuated by his very helplessness.

Despite these real difficulties in sharing the home of relatives and his disinclination to doing so, the patient is even more deeply disturbed if he is faced with the fact that relatives, particularly his children, do not want to take him. For no matter how realistic a basis children may have for not accepting their parent in their home, the patient, even while agreeing with the reality situation, reacts to the rejection which such a refusal implies, a refusal which accentuates the inadequacy caused by loss of health and independent status.

It is evident that the reality confronting some of the patients is a very depressing one indeed. In many instances, little can be done to alter the existing situation. We cannot make adequate provision where no resources exist. Nor can we make children love their parent where no love exists. All we can hope to accomplish, if we are to ameliorate conditions for the patient, is to give him sufficient substitute support to enable him to regain some of his lost feeling of worth as a person, to help him function to the best of his ability and with some degree of satisfaction, despite the limitations imposed from within and from without.

LOSS OF ECONOMIC SECURITY

Emotional difficulties in the area of interfamilial relationships are not the only ones the patient has to face upon discharge. Equally important is the problem of economic security. While some patients, seeing no visible signs of improvement and feeling little, if any, relief from symptoms, may question their readiness to leave the hospital, others, whose symptoms have subsided, may view discharge as an indication that they have improved to the point where they can return to normal living. The extent to which their expectations will be realized, however, will be determined not by their desires or ambitions or goals but by the nature of the illness, the extent of the continuing disease process, and the degree to which medical science has been successful in arresting it. Many patients hope, and have a right to hope, that a cure will arrive tomorrow. Even when eventual return to normal, or near normal, activity can confidently be expected, there still remains the need for a period of readjustment, with resulting loss of security in the immediate present and until such time as a level of optimum functioning can be achieved.

This feeling of insecurity is further aggravated by the fact that many of the patients come to the hospital following a prolonged period of illness, with time lost from work, extensive medical bills, savings exhausted, and the burden of accumulated debts which all this usually implies. Thus the specter of economic insecurity plagues many of the patients who fear a continuing inability to care for themselves and hence the need to become dependent on grudging relatives or the humiliation of applying for public assistance.

Not only the nature and extent of the illness, but also the type of work which the patient is trained to do will determine the degree to which his working capacity is impaired. Some patients can return to their previous employment; others may have to face a reduction in work capacity to a greater or lesser degree; still others may be confronted with the necessity of making a complete change in occupation. Whether a temporary period of adjustment or a more permanent alteration in his established pattern of living and working is involved, the patient may require skilled help if he is to make the necessary transition with a minimum of tension and some degree of satisfaction. Experience has taught us that in this, as in so many other instances, our understanding of the patient's previous pattern of adjustment is of inestimable value in our attempts to bring him to terms with the demands his condition imposes upon him. Whenever a change is indicated, the best results are obtained when preparation for any adjustment is instituted early, when the patient's own attitudes, desires, and plans for the future, as well as his objections to the proposed changes, are taken into consideration, and when he is given the responsibility of participating actively in planning.

DIFFICULTIES THAT CONFRONT CHILDREN

For many children suffering from prolonged illness, discharge from the hospital, while eagerly anticipated, is but the beginning of a new and often a difficult way of life. When the handicapping sequelae of illness are not visible externally, the child may look forward to resuming a life of activity and play with his friends, only to discover that he must confine himself to being an outsider, watching the activities of his former playmates but not participating in them.

Even for those who can approximate a more or less normal way of life with minimal restrictions, the adjustment may be a difficult one. Children wish to conform; they want to be exactly like other children and do exactly what other children do. Restriction of activities, no matter how minimal, is hard for them to accept. Even more difficult is the adjustment when the child's handicap is visible to others. The need to use crutches, or to wear braces, for instance, even though he is able to handle them adequately, or the need to attend a special school, sets him apart, singles him out as being "different" and, therefore, not so good as the others.

While little can be done to change the situation for many of these children, adequate preparation for discharge is as important as preparation for hospitalization. Provision of substitute satisfactions for those which their condition denies them can ease, at least to a degree, the adjustment which confronts them.

GRADUAL TRANSITION TO COMMUNITY LIVING

In our attempt to restore the patient with prolonged illness to maximal physical, mental, and social usefulness, it is important that he be given an opportunity to make the difficult readjustment from the dependency of hospital existence to independent community living gradually. A period of "gradual transition" during which the patient is expected to assume more self-responsibility, while being fortified with some measure of protection, is an ideal way to insure the best possible adjustment.

We have long been familiar with the use of a convalescent period for the restoration of sick people to normal living following an acute illness. How does this concept apply to sufferers with prolonged illness?

What do we mean by convalescence? The dictionary defines it as "a state of progressive restoration to health and strength after the cessation of disease." Since the very fact of chronicity precludes the cessation of disease and the restoration to health and strength, it is evident that this concept is inapplicable to the long-term patient. And yet, a period of gradual transition is essential to insure a return to maximal physical well-being and social usefulness.

The very fact of protracted hospitalization, more common among patients with prolonged illness than among the acutely ill, with its more complete separation from the outside world, would seem to argue for a more gradual process of readjustment such as is possible in a nursing home, devoted to such a purpose and no other and functioning under the supervision and control of a general hospital.

Among the advances made in the treatment of prolonged

illness is the recognition that the physician's recommendation that a "few weeks in a quiet place in the country, good food, and rest is all that the patient needs" no longer suffices. Nowadays, we are apt to think of the period immediately following hospitalization, not as an indication of the cessation of the interest of the hospital, but rather as another step in the hospital's total program of medical care.

Because this concept is comparatively new, there is a marked shortage of adequate nursing homes equipped to provide the type of care which is required. A recent survey indicates that

The Nation has about 23,000 nursing homes, homes for the aged, personal care homes and rest homes. They can accommodate less than 600,000 persons. Only 9,700 of these homes are staffed and equipped to give skilled nursing care and they have room for only 388,700 patients. At least half a million more beds are needed right now for long-term patients according to the total estimates of need made by the States. As life-spans continue to lengthen, as higher nursing home standards remove the dread which still prevents many older people from deciding to enter a nursing home, and as health insurance is extended to cover nursing home care, the demand for good nursing homes will grow apace.[1]

Not only is there a shortage of nursing homes, but the usefulness of the existing facilities is limited by the way in which they function. Lack of individualization; demand for strict adherence to established routines; an arbitrarily set limited stay; restrictive admission policies on the basis of diagnosis (including many prolonged illnesses), race, age, sex, or the need for special diets—all militate against their utilization in the best interests of the patient. It would almost seem as if those patients who are most urgently in need of such care are the ones most frequently excluded.

If patients are to derive maximal benefits from nursing home care, facilities for such care should be integrated into

[1] President's Council on Aging, 1963, *Federal Aid for Nursing Homes*, p. 1.

the over-all medical treatment plan center. In order to be used constructively it must be related to the individual patient, his needs and desires. Some patients may be miserable away from their family. For them this period, even under ideal circumstances, would represent only a prolongation of the period of separation. Others may see nursing home care as a means of continuing in a dependent role. For still others, the major advantage would be in the postponement of the necessity to return home and face the daily responsibilities of normal family life. There are instances where the depressing reality which awaits him in the world outside is so difficult to face that the patient looks upon his stay in the nursing home primarily as an escape. Recognizing that escape rarely solves the patient's problem, it devolves upon those responsible for his care to help him face and handle whatever difficulties he is likely to encounter.

The case of Mr. D. is an example of a patient who, quite understandably, sees his stay in the nursing home as a means of escape:

A man in his early thirties, Mr. D. was admitted to the hospital for a surgical procedure involving his spine. He was adjusting well and apparently needed no help from the social worker throughout his stay in the hospital. His recovery following surgery was uneventful.

One day Mr. D. approached the social worker with the statement that the doctor told him he could be discharged home shortly. Would it be possible to arrange to send him away for a few weeks so he could "rest up"? He thought that the country air would do him good.

In the absence of a medical recommendation for convalescent care, the worker, while agreeing that a few weeks in the country would be very pleasant, questioned whether there was any reason why he could not get a "rest" at home, perhaps spend some time in the park? In response to this question, Mr. D. described his home situation. He related with considerable bitterness that he, his wife, and their two children were living with the wife's parents. The home was overcrowded, there was little opportunity for privacy or rest. Moreover, Mr. D. did not get along with his father-in-law, and they had not spoken to each other for many months.

Just before Mr. D. entered the hospital, the family made application for an apartment in one of the housing developments and expected that an apartment would be available within a few weeks. He admitted that his request for convalescent care stemmed not from the doctor's recommendation but from his desire to escape from facing the intolerable home situation. He did not feel well enough to cope with the tensions and quarrels which he was sure would occur. If he could get away for a few weeks, then he would be able to go to his own apartment.

The worker agreed that the situation might indeed be difficult. She pointed out, however, that convalescent facilities are scarce and the chances of his being admitted slim. Furthermore, delays in securing apartments often occur. There was no guarantee that if he went away for a couple of weeks, he could then move to his own apartment. Could Mr. D. see what he could do to make the situation more tolerable at home? Mr. D. doubted whether any change could be brought about. However, he agreed that being reunited with his wife and children was something to look forward to. The knowledge that this was not a permanent arrangement and that it would not be long before they could move to their own apartment should make it easier to tolerate whatever discomforts would be involved, he agreed.

It is true that under existing conditions, the meager facilities available must be conserved for those whose medical condition makes such care essential. One might question, however, whether Mr. D.'s total welfare would not have been advanced if he had not been compelled to return to a situation so fraught with possibilities of friction and unhappiness.

PAUCITY OF CUSTODIAL FACILITIES

An entirely different set of problems confronts those patients who at the time of discharge from the hospital are suffering from permanent infirmities not amenable to continued medical treatment and have no home adequate for their needs. Unable to profit any further from the highly skilled and costly medical care provided by a modern hospital, they nevertheless will need the protective environment of an institution for a long time or, in some instances, even permanently. What is open to patients who can return neither to their own home nor that of relatives? Despite the tendency, so prevalent in the past, to regard prolonged illness as requiring primarily custodial care, it is a well-known fact that provisions for such care are inadequate to keep pace with the demand. This inadequacy, which applies to both public and private institutions, is being constantly aggravated by the rapid growth in the incidence of prolonged illness and the advances in medical science which keep people with such illness alive for longer periods of time.

It is difficult to estimate with any degree of certainty the number of available custodial institutions. While the term "custodial institution" usually refers to an institution which provides only shelter and personal care, in reality under this term are grouped nursing homes, homes for the aged, personal care homes, and rest homes. Patients suffering from prolonged illness can be found in any of these institutions, regardless of the type of care their condition may require.

Because of the general shortage of available beds, waiting lists are often long, and patients recommended for such care are sometimes kept waiting for months, sometimes for years. Even in New York City, which has the largest number of so-called custodial institutions in the country, the total bed capacity is admittedly inadequate. It is safe to assume that the situation is worse in other parts of the country. Since it may be difficult to make temporary plans pending admission, these patients often remain in the hospital, occupying urgently needed beds. When their turn comes, many are reluctant to enter these institutions, reacting with anxiety to the implication of hopelessness which the custodial nature of the institution connotes. Their reluctance can be easily understood if we keep in mind the type of care provided.

Many of the government-supported institutions, following the pattern of the old almshouses from which they evolved, have retained the squalid surroundings, the poor food, and the inadequate care characteristic of the former. Lack of interest on the part of the personnel, inadequate provision for leisure-time activity, and total absence of any program of even partial rehabilitation frequently reduce the patient to a vegetative existence and consequent deterioration. Because the patient's condition is considered to be "chronic," requiring a minimum of medical care, concomitant illnesses often go unrecognized, sometimes with disastrous results.

Because of the inadequate care supplied by the public custodial institution, large sections of the community find the privately owned nursing homes more acceptable. In reality, however, they frequently duplicate the undesirable features of the public institutions. Private facilities are also scarce, the waiting lists long. In addition, the cost frequently is prohibitive, and they are often no better equipped than the public homes to provide adequate care.

The most serious drawback, however, of many public and private institutions is their physical isolation and almost complete separation from centers of medical research and treatment. Thus, the patient is deprived of prompt and adequate medical treatment when he may need it most. What is equally important, from a long-range point of view, is that he is removed from the interest of those scientists who are concerned with new methods of treatment of prolonged illness. In addition, the physical distance means that the patient is deprived of frequent contact with friends and relatives, a contact which becomes doubly important because of his prolonged and sometimes even permanent institutionalization.

The increased demand for custodial homes has resulted

within recent years in a rapid expansion of private institutions with inadequate governmental supervision or control and an absence of mandatory standards. Consequently, we find that these institutions, operated for personal financial profit, vary greatly in physical facilities and personnel.

A survey conducted in New York State indicates that there has existed since 1944 "a limited system of inspection and certification of proprietary nursing homes [many of them custodial institutions] by local authorities (to provide) minimum standards for the care of persons the cost of which was borne indirectly from public funds," but no actual supervision.[2] In the absence of such supervision, it is to be expected that the commonly accepted standards, the financial resources of the proprietors, and the concept of what they consider to be a fair financial return will continue to be the deciding factors determining the type and extent of services rendered.

The situation has improved but little since this statement was made. The 1963 report issued by the President's Council on Aging states that "because of the shortage of nursing homes . . . . licensing requirements are often the minimum standards that will assure a patient's safety and comfort."[3]

In reviewing the available facilities, it must be mentioned that steps to remedy the situation were taken in New York City where in 1963 a Proprietary Nursing Home Code was established, enforcing both construction and operating standards. The latter are under the authority of the Department of Hospitals which enforces supervision of the medical standards, record keeping etc. As a result of these new requirements many marginal nursing homes have been forced to leave New York City.

There are a few voluntary "hospitals for incurables"

[2] New York State Department of Social Welfare, p. 2.
[3] President's Council on Aging, *Federal Aid for Nursing Homes*, p. 6.

where both the medical supervision and the physical facilities are more nearly adequate for the care these patients require. Their number, however, is so small and the waiting list so long that they fail to solve the problem to an appreciable degree.

It can thus be seen that the question, "Where do I go from here?" asked by many patients with prolonged illness is a very real one and that no easy answer has been found.

FACILITIES FOR CONTINUED MEDICAL CARE

Let us consider the second question uppermost in the mind of the patient when his hospitalization comes to an end: "Where do I get the medical care I still need?" There is no single answer to this question, for the type of care required is not uniform for all patients. Rather, it is determined by the patient's condition at the time he leaves the hospital. He may require the type of care which can be rendered on an outpatient basis, in a clinic or in the office of a private physician. He may have to remain in a custodial type of institution with a minimum of medical supervision. Or he may continue to need intensive medical and nursing care which can be given in his home, if he is able to carry the cost involved.

The provisions for patients who require custodial or nursing home care and the inadequacy of available facilities have already been discussed.

FACILITIES FOR OUTPATIENT CARE

For those patients who can maintain themselves in the community, whether in their own home, the home of a relative, or a substitute home, the outpatient department of the hospital or the office of a private physican are the two traditional avenues for continued medical care.

Some of the drawbacks of clinic care have been discussed earlier. However, we must not overlook the fact that attendance at a clinic attached to the hospital where the patient had been treated has certain positive values. The knowledge that all details of his condition are available to the physician treating him, so aptly expressed when the patient says "this doctor knows my case," the presence of personnel whom he knows and has learned to trust, the very familiarity of the hospital, give the patient some measure of continuity and security. How important this security in the familiar setting may be to some patients is well illustrated by the resistance shown when referral to a clinic nearer home is recommended. Many patients whose condition makes traveling to and from the clinic difficult, nevertheless show preference for this arrangement despite the physical strain involved.

It is important to remember that while continuation of medical supervision is essential to the adequate care of prolonged illness, such supervision is not without its threats to the patient. Implicit in the clinic visits is an ongoing reevaluation of the patient's condition. The fear of what such a reevaluation might reveal and the need for readjustment to medical recommendations are sources of ever present anxieties. Some patients become fearful when faced with a medical recommendation for increased activity. Having become accustomed to a limitation of activity, having been told over and over again that they must be careful and should "take it easy," they need considerable reassurance and interpretation that they are physically capable of assuming additional activity, no matter how limited. The return even to minimal activity means a slow and gradual process of overcoming the dependency encouraged during hospitalization and learning to assume some measure of responsibility once again.

Other patients, confronted with the doctor's recommendation for restriction of activity, need help to prevent them from undertaking more than their physical condition permits. Even the extremely dependent person who, it might be assumed, would welcome such a recommendation which satisfies his dependency needs, may react with anxiety to the implication that his phyical condition shows signs of deterioration.

Because of the nature of prolonged illness it often happens that reactivation of symptoms or an aggravation of the patient's condition necessitates rehospitalization. When this occurs, many patients are reassured by the fact that readmission to a familiar setting can be arranged without delay. We have found that the readiness of the hospital to readmit a clinic patient when the need arises, tends to lessen his anxiety and mitigates to some extent the feeling of rejection engendered by discharge.

While medical follow-up is an essential part of the treatment of prolonged illness, the outpatient department of the hospital is not the only source of continued medical supervision. Many patients return to the private physician who knew them prior to hospitalization. This arrangement is a satisfactory solution when the patient can afford the cost.

In view of the continuing disease process in many of the prolonged illnesses, and the consequent importance of continued medical supervision, it is indeed unfortunate that a large number of discharged patients do not follow through on systematic periodic check-ups either at a clinic or at the office of a physician. Many of them soon forget the doctor's recommendation and continue without medical attention until the next acute episode makes readmission to a hospital imperative. It is reasonable to assume that, given adequate medical supervision and attention to intercurrent illnesses, many readmissions could be avoided.

HOME CARE

Among the patients who have to face the problems of discharge is a group who neither require custodial care nor are well enough to depend solely upon outpatient care or occasional visits to a private practitioner. These are the patients who can remain at home but who continue to need active medical and nursing care and are unable to meet the expense. Even were it possible to build enough hospitals and maintain enough beds to accommodate this group of patients, hospital care would not necessarily be the answer to the problems they present. For the stage of their illness does not require the highly specialized facilities a hospital stands ready to provide, and the advisability of their remaining indefinitely in the hospital, with all that it implies, is open to serious question.

Until some twenty years ago, there were no organized facilities available for their care. The home care program at Montefiore Hospital in New York, initiated in 1947 and designed for the care of medically indigent patients in their own homes, was hailed as revolutionary, holding promise of influencing the total planning for future medical care of patients with prolonged illness. Within the first few years of its existence, the advantages of this program have been so well demonstrated that other hospitals have adopted similar programs.

The home care program was conceived as an extension of hospital care into the patient's home with the hospital continuing to carry full responsibility for his welfare and for the quality of medical care provided. Its purpose was twofold: to provide the patient with effective medical care in his own home; and, at the same time, to insure the most constructive utilization of available hospital beds.

This double purpose embodies the philosophy underlying the program. In it is implicit not only the recognition that hospital facilities should be available to the patients who need them, but also that, by the same token, a patient who can no longer profit by what the hospital has to offer should not occupy a hospital bed merely because other facilities are lacking. In line with this thinking, the decision as to whether a patient is to receive care in the hospital or at home was at no time based merely on administrative expediency or on pressure for hospital beds. Rather it was determined by a thoughtful consideration of the patient's condition and of what would best serve his interests, both medically and socially, at a particular stage of his illness.

It was recognized from the very beginning that the importance of social factors, so essential in any program of total medical care, assumes added significance with the patient's return home. By virtue of their day-by-day interaction, the effect of social, economic, and emotional problems of the family upon the patient and the impact of the patient's illness on the total structure of family living become even more direct and more important. In order to make medical care in the home effective, it becomes necessary to integrate it closely with simultaneous treatment of whatever social problems may arise, and to utilize to the utmost the constructive values and strengths inherent in family living. This close integration of attention to social factors as part of a total medical-social approach to the patient thus becomes the foundation on which a home care program must be built, influencing the selection of patients, the various services provided, and the evaluation of results obtained.

To insure the smooth functioning of the program, patients had to be selected on the basis of carefully established criteria—medical, nursing, and social. It can be readily seen that in the total planning it might be difficult to separate the determination of medical and nursing suitability from the social, for the very carrying out of the necessary medical and nursing care is inevitably affected by the social situation. In line with the avowed purpose of the program, it is essential that the physician determine the type of care required by the patient before any plans for home care can be entered into. While it is evident that neither patients whose medical condition requires hospitalization nor those who can receive adequate care on an outpatient basis, whether in a clinic or by a private physician, would be suitable subjects for home care, the decision needs to be a positive as well as a negative one. In other words, in thinking of posthospital care it is not enough to say that there is nothing in the patient's condition to prevent him from attending a clinic. It must be definitely determined that outpatient care is the best possible care for him at this particular time. Similarly, it is not enough to say that a patient no longer needs the specialized facilities of a hospital and can, therefore, be cared for at home unless we know that care in the home will serve his interests best.

One of the primary prerequisites for a home care program is the availability of a home to which the patient can return, whether it be his own home, that of a relative, or any other substitute home. The mere physical availability of a home, however, is not enough. Patients medically eligible for home care are frequently limited in the amount of activity they can undertake; sometimes they are confined to a wheel chair or are completely bedridden. It is essential, therefore, that there be someone in the home who is willing and able to take responsibility for helping the patient with his everyday needs. Nor is this all. Even the most comprehensive medical program, supplemented by home nursing care, cannot supply the twenty-four-hour-a-day attention which the patient requires, and the burden of such care inevitably falls upon family members. If unable to supply such care themselves, the family may require the help of home aids to relieve them of part of the physical burden involved.

Taking all these things into consideration, it is evident that, in order to be suitable and to make possible the rendering of medical and nursing care, the home must have at least a minimum of physical comfort. Yet, we have learned through experience that no arbitary set of standards can be established; nor can we impose our preconceived concept of what constitutes a desirable standard. The physical condition of the home, the economic status of the family, may not measure up to what we consider as satisfactory, but they may be vastly outweighed by the meaning the home has for the patient and the satisfactions he derives from his association with it.

Theoretically, for instance, it would seem essential that a certain amount of privacy would be a prime prerequisite to insure adequate medical care. And yet this is not always the case. As an example, let us consider the case of Mr. O.:

Mr. O. felt keenly his separation from home and during his hospitalization spoke frequently about his family. He looked forward with eagerness to the day when he would be able to return home.

When he was finally ready to leave the hospital, Mr. O. was overjoyed. It was evident, however, that he would continue to need a great deal of medical and nursing attention, the cost of which was beyond the family's meager means. The suggestion that the necessary attention could be provided under the home care program was welcomed eagerly both by the patient and the family members. The one factor, however, which seemed to present serious difficulty was the crowded condition of the home and the consequent lack of privacy. The patient needed a hospital bed, and the only space available for it was in the living room. Under these circumstances, the doctor questioned whether the patient would be able to secure the rest and quiet so necessary for him. However, because Mr. O. and his family were so eager for his return home and so willing to make whatever adjustments this demanded, it was decided to attempt the experiment.

It soon became apparent that had it been possible for Mr. O. to have a room for himself, it is questionable whether he would have been any happier at home than he was in the hospital. A forceful person, Mr. O. had previously been the undisputed head of his family. With the hospital bed in the living room, it was not long before he once again became the center of the life of the family and an active participant in all that transpired. The satisfaction he derived from this arrangement far outweighed the benefits of "rest and quiet" orginally prescribed for him.

While this may be an isolated instance, it confirms our belief, based on years of experience, that given a favorable home atmosphere, a stable social situation, strong family ties, a basic acceptance of the patient, and genuine concern for his welfare, even the drawback of what might be considered serious physical inadequacies can be overcome. As another illustration let us cite the case of Mr. T.:

A man in the late fifties, Mr. T. made his home with his wife and two sons, aged 26 and 13. At the time he was considered for home care, there was serious question as to the suitability of the home. Mrs. T. was not well and found it difficult to do the ordinary household chores. It was evident that the additional burden of caring for Mr. T. might be too much for her. The family income was inadequate, the only source being the 26-year-old son's marginal earnings.

However, Mrs. T., as well as the children, was eager to have the patient home. When the doubts as to the type of care the patient would receive were discussed with the family, the son assured us that the patient would get the necessary attention, and that he would assume full responsibility. Since he worked in the neighborhood, he would be easily available in case of emergency or to give injections. He had planned to look for other employment with better prospects for the future, but was willing to forego this for the time being. Having his father at home was more important—everything else could wait.

To assure that Mrs. T. would be relieved of some of the household responsibilities and be able to devote some time to her husband, arrangements were made for part-time domestic help to take the burden of the heavy household work off her shoulders.

The arrangement worked out satisfactorily. The patient received the necessary care, and the family was happy to have him at home.

If we keep in mind all the factors that must be taken into consideration to insure for the patient adequate medical care in the home, it becomes apparent that the decision should be made on the basis of a careful appraisal of the social and familial as well as the medical aspects of the situation. The social evaluation and the determination of social eligibility

thus become part and parcel of the total medical-social evaluation to answer the question: "Is home care the best possible
plan for this particular patient, for his family, and for the
community?"

Difficulties inherent in a home care program.—The description of the program clearly points up the advantages inherent in being able to secure adequate medical care in the
home. Nevertheless, it must be remembered that some patients may have difficulty in adjusting to a program so radically different in many respects from that in a hospital. Some
patients, accustomed to the dependency characteristic of prolonged illness and hospitalization, may fear the sudden resumption of more self-responsibility which a return home
implies. For these patients, the continued interest of the hospital personnel and the services given by the program mitigate, at least in part, the threat of too complete a separation
from the protection hitherto provided by the hospital environment. When the plan for home care is first discussed, patients may have reservations as to whether these services will
actually be available to them. Their sense of security is
strengthened only as they learn that their needs are met as
they arise, that the hospital and its facilities stand ready to
help them, and that they can return to the hospital if it becomes necessary.

Others find it difficult to accept the disappointment that,
despite their return home, the limitations imposed by their
illness persist, their activity is still limited, and they have to
continue under strict medical supervision. One of the most
difficult problems confronting a patient under these circumstances is the adjustment to his new status in the family
group. Aware of his weakness, his dependence, his inablity to
resume his accustomed role, he begins to question his ability
to retain the love and respect he previously enjoyed.

While a patient who is hospitalized for a prolonged period
is compelled to recognize that during his absence his responsi-

bilities have been taken over by someone else, he is, however, protected from the full impact such realization implies. The very atmosphere of the hospital, the patient's concern with the acuteness of his illness, his physical removal from the affairs of everyday living, and the social sanction of the dependence characteristic of illness, all tend to minimize his embarrassment at not being able to discharge his usual obligations, and blunt his appreciation of the full extent of the displacement which occurs.

It is one thing to accept a dependence which he considers as temporary and which can be ascribed to the peculiarities of the hospital setup. It is quite another for the strong man, the mainstay of his family, to witness his displacement in his own home in the day-to-day living. Few people are sufficiently flexible, sufficiently secure, to be able to adjust to prolonged dependency in their own home without help. The social worker's skill is needed here even more than in the hospital, for with the patient's return home a new set of problems comes to the fore. The very familiarity of the surroundings, the impact of everyday problems of family living, encourage a return to the traditional patterns of behavior and evoke reactions conditioned by years of habit.

Because people differ in their reactions to any life situation that confronts them, they also differ in their reaction to being incapacitated invalids in their home. Some are meek; they strive consciously or unconsciously to be the "good patient," a silent sufferer who gives no trouble at all. Others, resenting their incapacity, carry over their resentment to those in the environment who are well. This resentment may manifest itself in a need to control, a control which can be exercised either by complete helplessness, claiming all the time and attention of family members, or by a refusal to submit to the demands of the illness, being "no trouble to others," doing more than they are able, thus creating anxiety and apprehension in those around them.

The case of Mrs. P. is an illustration of this latter reaction:

A 29-year-old woman suffering from multiple sclerosis, Mrs. P. was discharged from the hospital when it was felt that she could no longer profit by active medical care. Upon her return home she insisted that she was able to get out of bed to attend to her personal needs. She could not "make a slave of her husband," she said. "He is doing enough without having to wait on me hand and foot." In reality, she was undertaking more than she could handle and often fell and hurt herself. Instead of relieving her husband of a burden, she was actually intensifying it. Mr. P. found that his sleep was never deep, as he was constantly watchful lest his wife attempt to get out of bed. After a while, his own physical condition was affected, and his business began to suffer.

Regardless of the degree of incapacity induced by the illness, the patient may expect that, the separation from family and friends having come to an end, the old pattern of family living will be resumed and he will automatically step back into what he considers his rightful place. Confronted by the limitations imposed by his physical condition, he may find that he is not able to regain the independence he had looked forward to at the point of discharge. He may discover, to his dismay, that he not only has to remain dependent on others for the physical care, but that the life of the family goes on around him as if he were not there.

How difficult the initial adjustment may be, despite the most careful preparation, is illustrated by the case of Mrs. V.:

A widow in her early sixties, Mrs. V. had been confined in the hospital for several months when the plan for discharge on home care was broached.

Prior to her illness, Mrs. V., a self-reliant, active woman, was the head of the household which she maintained for her working children. The prospect of returning home a semi-invalid confined to a wheel chair and dependent upon her children filled her with fear and apprehension.

Several months of intensive work by the social worker were

necessary before Mrs. V. would agree to the plan. During this period efforts were made to bolster Mrs. V.'s confidence in her ability to maintain herself in the home and to contribute leadership to the family group despite her handicap.

When she finally returned home, her first reaction was one of utter discouragement. She found herself faced with all the difficulties she anticipated and could see no way in which she could alter the situation. She felt that she contributed nothing to her family and was instead imposing a heavy burden on them. Rather than continue in this way, she said she would prefer to be sent to a "home for incurables." So intense was her reaction that it seemed at first that the home care plan would have to be abandoned and custodial placement arranged.

In an attempt to ameliorate the situation, Mrs. V. was visited frequently. Every slight evidence of progress was emphasized so that step by step her self-confidence was restored. With careful and consistent encouragement, Mrs. V. was able gradually to take on more and more responsibility, first learning to care for her own needs and later to assume part of the burden of house-keeping.

In view of the very real limitations imposed by the patient's condition, a sustained effort must be made to mitigate to some extent the patient's feeling of uselessness, his awareness of displacement in his own home, and to create possibilities for drawing him into the pattern of family living, no matter how minimal the responsibilities. What these responsibilities will be, will vary with each individual situation. They will be determined not only by the extent of the patient's physical capacity, but, more important, by the type of person the patient is, the meaning he holds for the family, what his illness and hospitalization meant to him and those around him, how much they are willing to forego in order to make the patient happy, the sacrifices they are willing to make in readjusting their lives to include the sick person. If our efforts on the patient's behalf are to be successful, we will need to draw upon and utilize to the utmost every possible

aspect of the family relationships and all the strengths inherent in the family goup.

It is important to recognize that the very services the
program is prepared to render can be a threat to the patient's
feeling of adequacy unless the main purpose of building a
constructive life for him is constantly kept in mind. Let us
consider one of the services, namely, provision of household
help, which is frequently necessary in order to carry out a
program of adequate medical care in the home. This service
can be of real benefit in relieving the family members of
heavy chores and thus giving them more time to devote to
the patient. Whether the service will achieve what it is
intended to do, or whether it will further aggravate the
patient's feeling of helplessness and uselessness depends, to a
great extent, upon how it is utilized.

For instance, outside help for a bedridden woman who is
deprived of her ability to fulfill the traditional role of a
mother may be an absolute necessity if good total medical
care is to be provided. But what happens to this woman,
incapacitated as she is, obliged to watch another woman take
over what once were her exclusive prerogatives, to watch the
children accept someone else and turn to this other woman
with their questions? The very fact that she is sick may
accentuate the patient's need to hold on to and control her
children and household. The harmful effect of the service,
whose need is recognized, can be reduced if an effort is made
to give the patient an opportunity to share in the over-all
responsibility for direction of the home and the children.
The children may have to turn to someone else for actual
help in doing things, but they can be taught to turn to the
sick mother with their questions, their problems, and their
joys. In the same way, allowing the patient to retain complete
control, with freedom to hire and fire the necessary domestic
help gives her the feeling that while she may not be able to
carry out the household duties herself, she is nevertheless

exercising her parental role. Instead of being a threat, the service can thus be utilized as a means of affirming the patient's worth as an individual and of showing what the patient can do in spite of the illness rather than concentrating on what she can no longer attempt to do because of it.

The story of Mrs. Q. is an illustration of what can be accomplished in making even a severely handicapped patient a useful and participating member of the family group:

Prior to her hospitalization, Mrs. Q. had been making her home with her daughter, son-in-law, and their two small children.

She was a valued member of the family group and assumed her fair share of responsibility in the care of the home and the children. When Mrs. Q. was ready to leave the hospital following an amputation, her daughter showed some resistance to accepting her mother back. The daughter explained that just before admission to the hospital the mother's care became so time-consuming that her own children were neglected. The patient was in pain, unable to care for herself, needed constant attention. Now, a chair-bound invalid, helpless, she would need even more attention. With a home, a husband, one child who was ill, how could she undertake the care of an invalid? Her husband too was concerned about her taking on this added responsibility, afraid that the strain would be too much for her and that the presence of the ailing mother would disrupt their family life.

The patient shared the daughter's feeling that the burden was more than anyone should be asked to assume. She did not want to make life harder for her daughter, who had always been good to her.

As they talked about the problem, it was evident that a strong bond existed between mother and daughter. The latter's resistance to the program stemmed not from a rejection on her part but primarily from a lack of knowledge as to the amount of care the mother's physical condition would entail, what she would be able to do for herself, and what contribution she could make to family living. Similarly, the patient's resistance to the plan was based, not on a lack of desire to return to her former home, but on a need to protect her daughter from a heavy burden.

Without minimizing the difficulties inherent in the situation, the patient's medical condition was carefully reviewed with emphasis on the prospect of continued improvement and the possibility of more activity in the future. The services the program stood ready to offer were gone over carefully.

As the story of Mrs. Q.'s previous role began to unfold, it became possible to point out not only what activities would have to be curtailed, but also what she could continue doing. She could help feed the children; she could read to them and sing the songs they so much enjoyed. At first she might not be able to prepare the meals, but she could teach the daughter the recipes for the old country dishes the family liked and missed. She could still sew and knit and mend.

As these discussions went on, the daughter began to see Mrs. Q. not merely as "a helpless invalid," but as the active, creative person she actually was, whose influence had permeated the life of the family for many years. The patient herself began to see that she would not merely be a burden, but could make a real contribution to those around her.

The initial adjustment was difficult. Despite all reassurances, the daughter tended to overprotect Mrs. Q., and the latter felt frustrated and useless. With continued help in the handling of specific problems as they arose, she was able to relax and to allow her mother more freedom of participation.

Several months after the patient's discharge, the daughter spoke enthusiastically about the arrangement and the help which the mother's presence in the home was to her. The patient too felt that she was being useful, was "earning her keep," and she "did not feel a burden anymore."

Family members, as well as the patient, may react to the strain of the patient's return home, even though they may have accepted the plan with enthusiasm when it was originally discussed with them. They may find that meeting the requirements of the patient's physical condition and, even more important, the need to provide continued emotional support, is more than they are able to sustain. If the home care program is to be successful, they may require the help of an experienced person who is able to help to relieve the tension.

Advantages of a home care program.—Mrs. Q. is only one of many patients cared for successfully on the home medical care program. The program has demonstrated that patients with prolonged illness can be successfully treated in the home and that, with proper safeguards, these patients not only are happier, but show definite physical improvement beyond what could have been anticipated. There can be no question that the return to familiar surroundings, eliminating as it does the strangeness of the hospital and the artificial routine of hospital life, the patient's happiness at being with his family, his feeling that he is not "put away" but is in a real sense an active and participating member of the family group, all contribute to his total sense of well-being and therefore to a more satisfactory response to medical treatment.

As social workers, dealing with people in trouble who come to us with problems in interfamilial relationships, we are in danger of emphasizing the problems and overlooking some of the positive forces in family life we can draw upon. We are likely to forget that family living not only creates problems for its members but is also a source of strength. In our culture, the family as a unit provides the best opportunity for growth and fulfillment, the place where the individual can best express his natural potentialities and satisfy his creative and emotional needs. Even when society apparently casts out an unproductive member, the family circle can be counted on to provide such loyal support, affection, sympathy, and understanding that, despite his handicap, the sick person can continue to participate in and guide the practical affairs of everyday living.

In an article describing the operation of the Montefiore Hospital home care program, the authors evaluate what the program can accomplish. In conclusion, they state:

The quality of medical care given Mr. S. was as good as that given him in the hospital, but to it was added the continued presence of those who loved him best and respected him most. Cures take less time this way, if only because the patient's struggle for life during his illness can be strengthened by a personal kind of medical attention in his own environement. Short of permanent cure, no patient can ask for more.[4]

The home care program has certain values, not only for the patient and his family but also for the medical practitioner who is interested in the implications of a program of total medical care. Dr. Martin Cherkasky, who directed the program for Montefiore Hospital for the first four years of its existence, states:

To the doctors on the program it has brought a new realization of the importance of social factors in disease. This is true of any disease. It is particularly true of long-term disease where the stress of illness brings about many changes in the relationhip of the patient to his family, both emotionally and economically. Montefiore Hospital in New York has not only made its scientific machinery available to patients who live miles from its walls, it has also begun to learn new reasons why a patient becomes sick and why his illness is prolonged.[5]

Though originally considered a revolutionary idea, home care is no a panacea or a total answer to the solution of the problem of prolonged illness. It is a new step in the treatment of a particular group of patients, though by no means limited to them, who until now have had little provision made for their care. It thus becomes a part of total medical care.

[4] Rosenfeld, Eger, et al., p. 116.
[5] Cherkasky, p. 163.

7

LEARNING TO LIVE WITH THE ILLNESS

O ur interest in the patient with prolonged illness and our concern with the provisions made for his care as evidenced in our discussion thus far are indications of the long road we have traveled in our attitude toward prolonged illness and its implications. The development has been a gradual one. Beginning with the medieval neglect and segregation of "incurables," we have moved to the concept of care of "chronic" patients as being merely the provision of a "shelter for the doomed," and have arrived, by slow stages, at the present-day appreciation of the need for integration of scientific medical care with social treatment of the patient as an entity, an integral part of the family group, and an indivisible part of the society in which he lives. Such a comprehensive approach embraces more than a concern with the patient's medical condition. Into it goes a consideration of the effect of the patient's medical condition upon his total life situation and of the way in which his social situation and emotional attitudes influence his ability to avail himself of the treatment medical science puts at his disposal.

INTEGRATION OF MEDICAL
AND SOCIAL TREATMENT

The present-day concept of total medical care, with its complete integration and treatment of the social as well as the medical problems can perhaps best be illustrated through the story of Paul Brown:

At 28, Paul Brown had already accumulated considerable experience with illness, hospitals, and doctors. He had become aware of vague joint pains and swelling and a general feeling of fatigue four years ago. These seemingly innocent symptoms gradually increased in intensity until, in fright, he sought out his family doctor who advised immediate hospital admission. This was the first in a series of admissions for Mr. Brown. In the four years he had spent many months in several hospitals, had gone South for his health, had exhausted his resources, and was still unhelped.

The social worker first came to know Mr. Brown after a thorough medical work-up had been completed, a definite diagnosis of rheumatoid arthritis of the spine and peripheral joints established, and treatment initiated in the arthritis clinic. At this point, he was referred by the doctor for a discussion of the medical regimen that had been prescribed for him. This was a six-point program which included complete bed rest except for weekly clinic visits, deep x-ray therapy, a high-calorie diet, gold-salt injections, and a back brace.

The actual medical recommendations formed the basis of a long and deepening casework relationship between the social worker and the patient. At first Mr. Brown denied his need for any help, although the toll his illness had already taken was apparent. Once a handsome young man, he was now thin and drawn, walked painfully, and could only get up from a chair with pronounced effort. He had been forced to give up a highly paid job as a furniture salesman and was now dependent on his family for financial help. Only when he found himself unable to purchase the back brace that had been medically recommended did he seek out the social worker and begin to use her services.

It was in his discussion of the brace that the patient first began to voice his confusion and desperation about his illness. Before he could bring himself to accept financial help with the brace, Mr. Brown had to be convinced that it would be of sufficient therapeutic value to compensate both for the change in his appearance it would create and the loss of independence it symbolized. The worker arranged for him to speak with the doctor, who clarified the medical necessity for the appliance, and he finally consented not only to obtaining it through the social service department but to wearing it as well.

The trust developed in this contact enabled the patient to seek the worker regularly for help with each step in the medical program, as it developed. Gradually, he began to express to her some of the deeper meaning that being sick held for him. Against the dreary background of his present situation, he sketched his former way of living, pointing out how much more satisfactory it had been when he had been able to get away from the home situation which, he hinted, was intolerable, and mingle with his many friends. He spoke of the fact that he had never taken his meals at home prior to his illness, and implied that facing his family at the table indicated to him forcibly his own inadequacies. Over and over again he expressed his rebellion at the present situation and attributed to the past all that was good and meaningful in living.

In an effort to alleviate the patient's difficult social situation, the worker, after consultation with the doctor, began to help him to make work and recreation plans.

It was the patient's body that first gave a clue to the fact that such plans were not meeting his real needs; for while he went along with all the planning and gave it verbal acceptance, his body negated the desire to get well which Mr. Brown consciously expressed. Despite the fact that he was coming in regularly for treatment and was apparently following instructions to the letter, he seemed to be going downhill rapidly. He himself noticed his failure to improve but seemed unable to express much anxiety about it or to articulate any dissatisfaction with the treatment.

At this point, the worker, more sensitive now to the possible psychosomatic factors in the situation, began to question in her own mind whether Mr. Brown really wanted to get well and to look for the possible sources of satisfaction that he might be deriving from his illness. It was clear that for this patient, illness had not brought the more usual gains of increased love and attention that cause many patients to cling to their symptoms. Instead, it had robbed him of whatever meager security he previously enjoyed, taking him away from his associates in the business and social world, subjecting him to the "humiliation" of coming to the clinic, depriving him of the handsome appearance in which he had taken so much pride, and bringing him acute physical pain and discomfort. Yet, given an opportunity to regain partially what had constituted his former sense of well-being, the patient resisted his chances to reenter his old world.

A review of the situation with the doctor brought to light the fact that Mr. Brown had never been able to overcome the idea that his present illness was caused by an old venereal infection, a fact which he had mentioned to the doctor when he first became ill and one which, the doctor indicated, still obsessed him. The doctor's reassurance that his present illness had nothing to do with the old infection seemed to have little meaning for the patient, who continued to discuss this possibility with the doctor although he was never able to mention it to the social worker. It seemed evident now to the worker that Mr. Brown might unconsciously be seeing his illness as deserved punishment for past indiscretions and could not, therefore, give up the illness before his guilt was eased. With help from the worker, he was able to articulate his conflict as involving a struggle between his wish to get well and his wish to stay sick, stating it in just those terms and asking the worker whether such a conflict is possible and how he might be helped to resolve it. Simultaneously, he moved in the direction of admitting his guilt about his illness, remarking that he had a "guilty conscience" which, he thought, might be making him sick.

Once he saw his problem in its entirety, as involving not only a set of physical symptoms but himself as a person, he was able to accept referral to a psychiatrist for help with his deep emotional problems and to involve himself in the recovery process.

Today, Paul Brown is holding down a sedentary job, seeing his friends regularly, once more enjoying life. He still wears a brace and walks with a limp and, once in a while, he experiences aches and pains. These symptoms no longer, however, cloak his resentment, his guilt, his insecurity. They merely indicate that he has a prolonged illness with which he has learned to live.

One may rightfully question how much physical improvement Paul Brown would have shown had his problem been attacked from the physical standpoint alone. It is safe to assume that the patient's inability to follow the medical recommendations so essential for his welfare would have annulled all the benefits of the counsel given him. For this inability did not stem from a lack of intellectual understanding to be overcome by reasoning and interpretation, but rather had its roots in deep-seated emotional difficulties of which he was but vaguely aware and with which he needed skilled help. It was only as he saw how his inner difficulties stood in the way of his recovery, and as he received appropriate help with these difficulties, that he was able to take the next step toward better health. The improvement shown by this patient can be ascribed not to the painstaking and excellent medical care alone, but to the integrated attack on his medical and social problems, to the individualization of the patient, and to the fact that the professional team was acutely aware that they were treating not "a case of arthritis" but "Mr. Paul Brown who has arthritis."

Paul Brown is but one of many patients with prolonged illness in our world today. The problems he poses for both the medical and social work professions may be duplicated in hundreds of cases. No one case, however, can adequately portray the numerous problems which prolonged illness creates, their manifold ramifications, or the various ways in which they can be treated. Just as we have learned that we cannot treat "a case of arthritis," we are beginning to learn that we cannot treat "a case of prolonged illness." In every instance, we treat not an illness but an individual. What our treatment will be is determined not only by our knowledge of the disease process, the physical effect it has on the patient, and the degree of incapacity it produces, but equally by our understanding of what the illness means to the particular individual, what his emotional needs are, and what help he may require to reconcile the demands of these needs with the reality his illness imposes. We have come to recognize that prolonged illness is not an isolated factor in the life of the patient. Rather, it becomes part of his whole life experience with roots in his past and significance for his future. Whether the patient is to remain confined to his bed in an institution, or can return to his home as an invalid, or even be able to function more or less independently; whether the need is for constant, fairly intensive medical supervision, or merely periodic check-ups, the illness remains with him and he must learn to live with it. If the increased skill of medical science in arresting the disease process and prolonging life is to be truly meaningful to the patient, we, the professional personnel caring for him, must be prepared to help him see that the restrictions imposed by the illness and the handicap which it may leave in its wake do not necessarily mean that he must give up everything that makes life worth living. With due regard to the necessary limitations and with a watchful eye for danger signals, the patient can and must be helped to learn to use that part of himself which remains unharmed.

As actual experience demonstrates again and again, attention to the patient's social and emotional problems bears rich returns in his better response to the medical treatment provided; and as the medical man sees these beneficial effects in his own work with patients, it is slowly, but consistently, changing his attitude toward patients with prolonged illness and the goals of all-inclusive medical care for them.

Whereas previously the focus of attention was the pathological condition, we now see the focus shifting to the person who has the illness and who, in the process of having his medical needs attended to, may lose what is equally important to him, namely, the sense of security he has had in his job, his family, and his social relations. For many years, the emphasis has been primarily on the alleviation of pain, the arrest of the disease process, and the postponement of a fatal outcome. The question which has been troubling many thoughtful persons is whether the arrest of a disease or the prolongation of life is, or should be, the single goal of medical science, or whether it carries with it an obligation to provide some assurance that this longer existence will be a fuller, more satisfying one. The birthday wish of a "long life and a happy one" takes on new significance.

The slogan of the *American Journal of Gerontology*, "To add life to years, not just years to life," might just as appropriately become the watchword for those of us who are concerned with the patient who suffers from a prolonged illness. Unless this is done, both the present and future accomplishments of medical science might well become anything but a blessing to those whom they are designed to help. This point of view was expressed in an address delivered at graduation exercises of the New York Medical College:

As the science of medicine moved deeper and deeper into our medical schools and our hospitals, the art of medicine was pushed further and further out of them. If we are to use this new scientific knowledge for the best interests of our patients, we must realize that science and art, like the scales of justice, must be perfectly balanced.[1]

Such a point of view, extensively adopted, would influence our treatment of the patient with prolonged illness from the very first day we come into contact with him, extending throughout his hospital stay and beyond, for as long as we continue to accept responsibility for the treatment of his medical condition.

THE MEANING OF TOTAL MEDICAL CARE
TO THE PATIENT

To the patient, such a changed approach may mean the difference between life and death. We know that in the past many a patient with a "chronic" illness died not from his

[1] Ravdin, p. 23.

chronic condition, but from an intercurrent illness which was often disregarded because of the overwhelming hopelessness of the primary diagnosis. Nowadays, the chronicity of the disease, the degree to which it has progressed, or the poor prognosis are no longer allowed to blind the medical practitioner to the possible presence of concomitant illnesses and the need to treat them. Even the old concept of "making the patient as comfortable as possible until the end comes" takes on added importance. Recognizing that a dangerous illness may transmit fewer distress signals than minor physical ailments, the doctor begins to appreciate that treating the aching foot, the ingrown toenail, the infected tooth or finger, may bring to the seriously sick person a measure of comfort out of all proportion to the seriousness of the presenting symptom or to the extent of medical help required.

Little by little the rigid differences in the approach to the treatment of acute and "chronic" patients are being abolished. The doctor who sees the sequelae of an acute illness in the patient with prolonged illness cannot escape the realization that it is essential to bring to the care of such a patient the same scientific approach that characterizes his attack on acute illness. The very challenge inherent in the possibility of preventing the development of chronicity of itself calls for an acceleration in the pace of diagnostic study and treatment. The recognition that the longer the disease is allowed to progress, the slimmer the chances for improvement, brings with it the conviction that the benefit of all the hospital facilities and the accumulated medical experience is as much a "must" in the treatment of the patient with prolonged illness as it is for the acutely ill one. As interest in the treatment of this group of patients increases, there inevitably appears evidence of a growing concern with the more far-reaching implications of prolonged illness, its causes, effects, and means of prevention.

If the awakened interest in, and understanding of, the effect of interrelation of the patient's emotional, social, and medical problems is to be of value, it must be translated into actual practice. First and foremost, it imposes an obligation to be constantly aware that no matter how serious the illness or how poor the prognosis, this fact in and of itself does not rob the patient of his status as a functioning, living being with the same rights which he enjoyed while well.

What are some of these rights? How do they relate to the person who is sick? What can be done to help preserve them?

HIS VALUE AS AN INDIVIDUAL

Basic among these rights is the right of the sick person to be treated as an individual. Once this becomes an accepted and integrated concept, the recognition of his other rights will necessarily follow. Illness per se does not change the person. The fact that "people" have become "patients" does not alter the fact that they remain "people," each of them an individual with differing backgrounds, differing ways of re-acting to what happens to him; and for each the illness may have different implications. Each one of them is not merely "a sick person" but a person who, in addition to his illness, has needs, desires, aims, purposes, and aspirations, has likes and dislikes, attitudes, moods, and feelings, who remains the product of all the forces that have influenced and fashioned him. His illness does not reduce him to the status of "the occupant of the bed in the right-hand side of the ward," or "that leg in the bed near the window." Nor does he become one of an anonymous mass, "the sick," whose very illness makes them different from "the well." He not only remains an individual in his own right, but also continues to be part of the society and the culture in which he lives and to respond to its customs, mores, and demands.

Illness, and particularly prolonged illness, does not lessen the patient's need to play the role which he feels society imposes upon him. What it does, is to give rise to frustration by pointing up sharply and unmistakably the irreconcilable discrepancy between what he considers his duties and goals to be and the realization of his utter inability to meet them. The resulting feeling of helplessness and the anxiety to which it gives rise demand from those concerned with the patient's care an extra measure of understanding, acceptance, and recognition of his value as a person.

HIS STATUS AS A MEMBER OF THE FAMILY

No one will dispute the statement that "the feeling of being accepted and considered worthy is one of the most potent forces of building inner strength and equips one to deal with life's difficulties." [2] Few life situations create such difficulties as those which confront the patient hospitalized for a prolonged period of time and, consequently, in few instances is the need to build the person's inner strength more essential. Removed from his accustomed surroundings and usual sources of satisfaction, subjected to the anonymity of hospital existence and the dependence imposed by his illness, the patient needs acceptance and recognition not only from the professional personnel concerned with his care but, even more important to him, from members of his immediate family group.

In our society we have accepted the concept that adulthood means independence—social, economic, emotional. It is through the maintenance of such independence that the normal adult gains status in his own estimation and in the eyes of those who form his circle. There is no rigid definition of what constitutes a satisfactory adult adjustment, but let us

[2] Woodward, p. 306.

consider the most commonly accepted standard. Usually, independence and status are achieved by the adult through the traditional role of breadwinner or homemaker. These assure for the individual approval and esteem from other members of the family and, once assured, are then reinforced by the more subtle and less tangible contributions of spiritual values they bring to family living. For both the breadwinner and the homemaker the discharge of these duties becomes the *raison d'être*—without them they are left adrift with a feeling that they do not count, that they have lost their right to a voice in the family council and to the love and respect they previously enjoyed.

So far as the breadwinner is concerned, the society in which he lives expects him to assume the responsibility for the family's economic welfare, and anything that interferes with the discharge of this responsibility becomes a threat to his adequacy, making him feel that he is less of a person because of it. Frustration, despair, or guilt are the usual concomitants. Any illness and hospitalization necessarily interrupts the patient's active participation in family living and discharge of family duties. Prolonged illness with its long separation carries with it the implication of a more permanent break of family ties and responsibilities and, consequently, a threat to his sense of belonging.

Thus, the patient afflicted with an illness of long duration, faced with the prospect of a prolonged cessation of his earning capacity, and the growing fear of its continuing indefinitely, is besieged not only by the worry as to what will happen to his family financially, but by the threat that his inability to provide will affect his standing with them. How far such a concern is realistically valid and justified can be answered only in the light of each individual situation, for a great deal depends on the strength of existing family ties. The threat, however, is real to all patients, for it is to members of his family that the individual looks for approval, love, and respect. The breadwinner's ability to hold a job, the fact that he is the provider, carries with it a feeling of competence, assurance, and authority. When the ability to provide is taken away, the inner feeling of the right to exercise authority goes with it. When a family needs to look for other sources of support, the breadwinner feels not only his own inadequacy but also the social stigma attached to it.

If we are to help the patient combat this feeling of inadequacy and the detrimental effect if produces, it becomes necessary to make him see that the preservation of his status does not depend entirely upon his ability to provide and that it can be maintained successfully through the quality of his relationship to the other members of the family, his interest in them, and their dependence upon him for advice and guidance. In order for the patient to be able to maintain his sense of belonging and his conviction of his own value, it is essential that he continue to make some contribution to family living. Even though his financial contribution is, of necessity, interrupted, he can be helped to continue his role by being consulted about matters affecting the family and by being involved in planning for them. With the realization that his value to family members goes beyond economic support, and that it can be maintained despite the withdrawal of his contribution, he will have less reason to fear the cessation of his earning capacity. In fact, in the light of the absence of his monetary contribution, the need of the family to turn to him for help in planning will assume added importance and will enhance and strengthen his feeling of worth and prestige. How this can best be accomplished, will be determined by the particular set of circumstances in each individual situation. The cases of Mr. R., Mr. W., and Mrs. Q., previously cited, are illustrations of what can be done when the concern for the patient as a person is uppermost in the mind of those dealing with him.

The woman as the homemaker also needs to feel that her

importance and share in family living are not totally destroyed by illness, by the long separation, or by the need to delegate to others the actual performance of her duties. To what lengths a patient may go to assure herself that she is missed by her family and that her absence makes an impression on their lives is well illustrated by Mrs. H.

Though she was critically ill and in severe pain, Mrs. H.'s only topic of conversation was her concern about the care of her 5½-year-old child during her absence. Since there was recognition of how important this was for her, Mrs. H. was involved in planning for the little girl's care. Arrangements were made for a trusted relative to stay in the home and look after the child.

After a six months' period of hospitalization, it was possible to arrange for Mrs. H. to see the child. She was pleased to see that the little girl looked well, had gained weight, and seemed happy and contented. As she told about the visit, Mrs. H. said that it made her feel better to know that all was going well. Now, she too would be able to relax and begin to think about herself and what she could do to speed recovery.

But, she added, the child had a slight cold. "If I had been at home, she would not have come down with a cold; I would have known how to shield her." As Mrs. H. talked about it she could admit that while she was "glad that all was well, it is hard to accept that all can be well without my being there." It was even a relief and satisfaction to her, she acknowledged, that the child had a cold, for it demonstrated that others could not give her little girl the same type of attention that she herself could.

Conscious of his inadequacy, the patient is acutely aware of any change in family attitudes, whether these be expressed in pity or through his relegation to a secondary place. In the light of the new understanding of the importance of the patient's attitudes and their influence on the results of medical treatment, it becomes the responsibility of the medical team to convey to family members their own feeling of the patient's worth as an individual. Such a conviction, when shared with the family and accepted by them, is as powerful a force for the patient's well-being as is penicillin or streptomycin in the hands of the physician. All the positive and health-provoking forces inherent in family living can then be drawn upon to fortify the patient, provide him with a real source of satisfaction and an incentive to continue his fight for life.

HIS STATUS AS A MEMBER OF SOCIETY

Carried one step further, this right of participation in family living is inevitably extended to the wider social circles surrounding the patient—his friends, his neighbors, and the community of which he is a part. Within these circles his value is even more likely to be judged by the extent of his self-sufficiency and economic independence or the lack of it; for the contact is more tenuous and precludes the formation of the more intimate associations of family living and the values such associations often bring to the fore. Recognition that the patient has a right to as full a life as his condition permits, carries with it a recognition of his right to companionship, recreation, and a sense of contributing to society within the limits prescribed by his illness, for all these are essential parts of a full life.

Unfortunately, this is a condition which is frequently difficult, and sometimes impossible, to achieve when the illness, necessitating long hospitalization, removes the patient from his day-by-day social contacts. The longer the hospitalization, the more constricted becomes his circle of companions. As the period lengthens, outside visitors, with the exception of very close members of the family, diminish, and the patient is confined more and more to the companionship of other patients, a companionship not of his own choosing. His ability to contribute to the life of the larger community may be drastically reduced, or even vanish completely. In addition, the demands of the illness, the constant preoccupation with self, serve to constrict the patient's sphere of interests.

As the patient's outside interests and associations lessen,

the limited world of the hospital takes the place of the larger world outside; the life of the hospital becomes a reproduction in miniature, within the limits imposed by the illness, of what his life was before the illness. It is indeed true that " 'misery likes company' is a perverted form of the gregarious instinct in hospital wards." [3] This continued preservation of the gregarious instinct is of inestimable value to the patient who has to remain within the confines of a hospital for a prolonged period of time. It enables him to find within this restricted community some substitute for the satisfactions he previously enjoyed in his social contacts. Here the strong, independent person, accustomed to having others lean on him, can still find some satisfaction in playing a similar role by "adopting" another patient whom he helps and advises, while the inadequate, dependent person can derive the satisfaction he needs by allowing himself to be "babied" by any fellow patient who shows an inclination to do so.

Nothing can give a better indication of the patients' interests and concern than can be obtained by attention to their behavior in the hospital and the topics of their conversations. There is, of course, the common bond of illness, leading inevitably to a discussion of symptoms and their treatment, of the doctors, nurses, and others with whom they come into daily contact, of the general happenings in the hospital. But above all else, the conversations center on a nostalgic recital of their past achievements and successes. Such discussions show all too clearly the patients' inability to accept their present limitations and their fear that illness robs them of their dignity. The inability to maintain their previous competence is to them a sign of failure and personal disintegration. To offset the daily evidence of his helplessness, the patient needs the reminder of a more satisfying past which helps him to bolster his ego and gives him the feeling that his past achievements are a measure of his true worth. Therefore,

[3] Bluestone, "These Administrative Axioms," p. 60.

the recital of his past accomplishments, regardless of their level, has value for him in and of itself. This value is reinforced if the patient's own evaluation of himself is accepted by others, particularly by people who are well, active, and useful. Such recognition not only helps him to overcome the feeling of worthlessness engendered by the illness, but serves as a demonstration that the illness does not deprive him of status, his worth, the love of those nearest him, or the respect of others in his environment.

HIS RIGHTS AS AN ADULT

The threat to the patient's feeling of his intrinsic worth is further reinforced by the humiliation of being dependent upon others for his daily care, of needing help where he previously was self-sufficient. Unfortunately, this dependence encourages in those ministering to his needs an inclination to treat him as a child, an inclination which is fostered by the childish mode of behavior to which patients frequently revert. If our obligation to protect the rights of the patient as an individual is not to go overboard, we must at all times keep in mind that what strikes us as childish behavior may be but the way in which the patient expresses his needs. The patient's peevishness and resentment of the hospital discipline may be his way of denying his illness; his demands for attention, a device to convince himself as well as others of his importance. His emphasis on symptoms and his apparent resistance to medical care may be expressions of an unconscious need to hold on to his illness and thus to avoid facing the reality which awaits him in the world outside. Unless we understand the roots from which such behavior springs, we may accept the seemingly irresponsible and immature behavior at its face value, which would make it difficult to remember that we are dealing not with a child, but with an adult who has a right to expect that he will be treated as such.

As part of his right to being considered an adult, the

patient has a right to know what is being done for him and why, to express opinions, and to use judgment in making decisions which ultimately will affect his entire future life. Acknowledging the patient's right to exercise such judgment implies a willingness to grant him the right to accept or reject help even when the medical situation demands drastic action and the help offered is the only means to improve his condition or even save his life. In view of our more intimate knowledge of the implications of such a refusal and our genuine desire to be of help, this concept is often difficult to accept and even more difficult to carry through to its logical conclusion. The more serious the procedure, the more important the consequences, the more difficult it becomes for us to stand by and allow the patient to reject it. For instance, when we know that by refusing surgery the patient is risking his life, that he is in reality determined on committing suicide, the temptation is strong to exert pressure "for his own good." And yet, if we subscribe to the concept of self-determination, to the conviction that any individual has a right to remain master of his own destiny, this should apply to the sick as it does to the well. The decision must be left to the patient as long as he is able to make a decision. If we are to be of real help in such a situation, we must remember to take into account the fact that different individuals react differently and that at no time can we really put ourselves in another person's shoes. What appears to us to be not only a reasonable but an important procedure may represent to the patient a threat more real than the illness itself, a threat which he may be unable to face.

Does this mean that no help can be given the patient in arriving at a desirable decision? On the contrary; we can help if we try to understand the reasons behind the refusal and to weigh these reasons carefully and with due regard for the patient's feelings. By our very recognition of his inalienable right to make the final decision, once all the reasons behind the decision are clearly understood; by showing our respect for his decision, no matter what it is; and by asserting our belief in his ability to decide on an adult responsible level, we can, and often do, encourage responsible behavior and influence the decision. The ability to withhold judgment, to avoid pressure by imposing our own point of view, requires the highest degree of skill and an uncompromising respect for the rights of the individual.

There was Anna X., for instance:

Mrs. X. was referred to the social worker when she threatened to leave the hospital against medical advice when there was a recommendation for chest surgery. In the opinion of the doctor, it was the only course open to arrest the spread of tuberculosis and to save the patient's life.

The worker found Mrs. X. disturbed, anxious, and tense. As if to avoid further discussion of the subject, the patient immediately informed the worker that she fully realized the step recommended was sensible, logical, and for her own good. She had decided against the operation, though she was fully aware of the implications of her refusal and the risk involved. Assuming that the worker was there to make her change her mind, she defiantly stated: "You cannot sell me the idea. That is what you are here for, isn't it?"

At first she found it difficult to believe that no pressure would be exercised to make her change her mind. She only half listened as the social worker emphasized that her only objective was to help Mrs. X. see clearly the reasons for and against the recommended step and to extend such assistance as might be necessary to carry out the plans which Mrs. X. had outlined for herself.

It was some time before Mrs. X. was able to accept the fact that the worker really meant what she said when she assured the patient the ultimate decision was hers to make. Convinced that no pressure would be brought to bear on her, Mrs. X. was able to relax and to verbalize some of the motives behind her resistance. She began to discuss her conflicting emotions, the various aspects of the problem, and to raise questions not about the decision itself, but about what made the decision so difficult.

At no time was an attempt made to make her change her mind. She was left with the feeling that she was primarily the one who had to face the operation and what it implied and, consequently, the one who had to decide what she wanted to do. The worker pointed out, however, that despite having made her decision, the patient did not appear happy with it. This too was understandable, the worker said. Presented with the necessity for a serious operation, it was normal that Mrs. X. would want and not want it at the same time, would fear what the consequences would be in either case.

As these discussions proceeded, and with increased confidence in the social worker's interest in her, Mrs. X. abandoned her previously repeated stand that under no circumstances would she agree to an operation. She began to talk about what the problems would be "should I decide to be operated."

The root of the difficulty in which this patient found herself and which she needed freedom to work out for herself was clearly revealed when she said: "Should I ever agree to the operation, I will want it because I want it, and not because I am being forced into it either by circumstances or by another person."

It took two months before Mrs. X., of her own accord, decided to undergo the necessary surgery. During this period no pressure was put on her. Over and over again, she was made to feel that we understood her hesitancy and that we were there to help her no matter what her final decision might be. At the end of that time, having settled the question in her own mind and having arrived at an independent decision, Mrs. X. approached the operation with a real conviction that it was the best thing for her, with faith in the outcome, and with only a minimum of normal anxiety.

The worker's approach to Mrs. X.'s problem, her willingness to stand by, no matter what decision the patient finally made, not only enabled this patient, as it does others in similar situations, to profit by the available medical care, but, also conveyed to the patient the feeling that she had the final word in what was going to happen to her. Under these circumstances, the patient ceases to be merely a passive recipient of a decision imposed on her from without and becomes an active participant in making and carrying out her own decision. How much this can mean to a patient, Mrs. X. indicated all too clearly.

As we look into the reasons underlying resistance to treatment and inability to make a decision, we find that they are frequently due to the patient's lack of authoritative knowledge of what the procedure implies, the reasons for it, and what can be expected as a result of it. Unfortunately, a busy physician all too often does not share such information fully with the patient. Experience has shown, however, that given such sharing, resistance diminishes and often vanishes:

A young woman came to the hospital with a slight swelling in her breast. She wanted to "make sure that it was nothing serious." The doctor decided to operate, but before going through with the operation he asked the patient to sign consent for a radical mastectomy, should it be indicated.

Despite the suspicions which originally brought the patient to seek medical opinion, the knowledge that "it might be serious" came as a shock—as it almost always does. The patient's initial reaction was a flat refusal. She could not understand why she needed to give consent for such a simple procedure.

After the reasons for the patient's refusal were explained to the doctor, he took the time to talk with her at length. He explained the nature of the proposed operation and pointed out the inadvisability of a double incision should it be found necessary to have the breast removed.

It is true that the explanation, no matter how carefully given, could not eliminate the threat inherent in the proposed procedure. The value of the explanation lay, primarily, in the fact that the patient knew why the procedure was necessary and what she could expect from it. As a result, her decision was made on the basis of knowledge and without the antagonism which an imposition of someone else's will frequently arouses.

These two instances illustrate the successful outcome of thorough discussion and freedom of choice in influencing the patient's decision. We have found through experience that while this cannot always be achieved, a discussion of pros and cons invariably helps to relieve the patient of his feeling of helplessness as he realizes that we admit his right to full knowledge and to a final decision based on such knowledge.

Sometimes the procedure advocated is not so serious as surgery but has, nevertheless, serious implications for the patient's health and welfare. For instance, strict adherence to a diet frequently presents stumbling blocks and is a source of irritation to hospital personnel and of complaints by the patient. Food habits are deeply ingrained, difficult to change. Where separation from the family is acutely felt, unfamiliar and unpalatable foods accentuate the separation. All too often, patients restricted to an unpalatable diet find a way to indulge their craving for more familiar and tastier food, no matter how strictly they are supervised.

On the other hand, a thorough explanation as to the need for the diet and securing the patient's cooperation in this phase of the treatment bear rich recompense. It not only eliminates the practice of circumventing the doctor's recommendations, but makes the patient a strong ally who understands the reason for the regime and helps in carrying it out, even when there is an opportunity to defy the order:

Tommy, a 14-year-old boy, was quite obese, and a reduction of weight was an essential part of his treatment. Tommy was given a thorough explanation of this phase of his treatment and the effect of the diet on his physical condition. His interest was enlisted in assuming the responsibility for charting his intake of food and his weight. As a result, he was not only able to assume complete responsibility for the faithful carrying out of the doctor's recommendations but could withstand the pressures brought upon him by his anxious mother who, in her eagerness to make up for all the deprivations he suffered, urged some of the forbidden delicacies upon him.

It is true that the extent of our ability to help is often limited by the patient himself and by his willingness and capacity to use help. This, in turn, is influenced by his intellectual capacity, by the stage of the illness, and the degree of mental damage created by it. In some terminal stages the ravages of illness dull the patient's capacities to an extent where active participation and a logical choice of alternatives become impossible. However, even in terminal stages the patient has a right to expect that he be treated as a living being as long as he lives and that he be given the right to decide how the life left him is to be lived. With this one exception our ability to be of assistance is limited only by our own feelings for patients as people and our respect for the individual and his rights.

HIS WORTH IN THE FACE OF PHYSICAL DETERIORATION

All the problems encountered in the handling of sick people are heightened when the patient realizes that, despite lengthy hospitalization and intensive medical treatment, he is not getting any better. As he feels himself going downhill he begins to doubt that he will ever get better and to fear that death is imminent. What can be done to help the patient in the face of such overwhelming hopelessness is a real challenge to all concerned with his welfare.

In this, as in other situations, it is important to remember that no two people react in the same way to any circumstances, not even to the universal fear of death. One patient comes to mind who, having intellectualized all his life experiences, also approached the problem of dying in intellectual terms, accepting death as a natural part of life, drawing strength from a review of his past achievements and satisfying experiences, continuing his intellectual activities and philosophical approach to the very end, and thus living to the last in the way life had meaning for him.

It is not often that a patient can intellectualize the experience in this manner. Many do not even dare to talk about their fear that they might die, the intensity of the fear itself making it difficult for them to discuss it openly. Often it is only as we learn to listen to what lies behind the spoken word that we are able to hear what the patient is trying to say. It is then that we begin to understand that by discussing the death of others, the patient is, in reality, voicing his own fears and asking for reassurance that this will not happen to him. Others give vent to their frustration and helplessness through complaints or aggressive behavior, as if by asserting themselves they attempt to negate the approaching dissolution of the ego which death implies. There are still others who react with a denial of the importance of what is happening to them. "What does it matter?" they ask. Every one of these attitudes requires an understanding of the meaning of death to the patient and an ability to face the problem with him on his own level.

Even when the patient wants to talk about his fear of dying, he finds few who are willing to listen to him. This is not surprising. Fear of death is inherent in all of us; it is inherent in the very process of living; it is part of the equipment with which we are endowed for self-preservation. Under pressure of their own fear of death and their concern for the patient, friends and relatives find it difficult, if not impossible, to allow him to talk about it. They attempt to escape what is to them an unbearable prospect by a pat on the back and by telling the patient that he is talking nonsense and that he will soon be well again. Well-meaning as such reassurance is, it carries little conviction in the light of what the patient knows to be true. The denial of what he is trying to convey means to the patient a disregard for what he feels, for what he says, and therefore a denial of himself as a reasoning person.

Faced with an overwhelming reality, there is little that anyone can do to eliminate the depression, the fear that usually accompanies it. There is no single formula that will dispel this ingrained fear of death. However, we can help the patient derive some measure of comfort if we can devise ways and means to maintain his inner conviction that the deterioration of his physical condition in no way affects his importance.

It is to the professional team caring for him that the patient has a right to look for help in this as in other situations connected with his illness. Unfortunately, the professional personnel too are handicapped by their own fear of death. In addition, the medical practitioner, faced with a situation over which he has no control, which he can neither alter nor alleviate, is brought face to face with his own inadequacy. The natural reaction is to avoid facing it, either by resorting to the pat-on-the-back technique or by actual physical escape. Neither the running away nor the denial of the reality is helpful to the patient, for it merely intensifies his anxiety and leaves him alone with his problem. If we can learn to listen to the patient speak of his fear of impending death, neither running away from it nor denying it, that in itself may be rendering a service of real value. By staying with the patient, we not only give him an opportunity to vent his feelings, but at the same time we affirm our regard for him as a person, our respect for what he is trying to tell us, and our understanding of, and sympathy with, his feelings. As was pointed out earlier in this book, the medical profession is gradually changing its point of view as to how this problem is to be met. It is to be hoped that under their leadership other members of the hospital team will also adopt a different attitude.

There are many more tangible ways in which we can help the patient maintain his feelings of remaining a living human being who still matters. This includes the provision of physical comfort and medical and nursing care, no matter how far the disease has progressed or how unfavorable the outcome. These services, elementary and essential as they may appear, are not always forthcoming in a busy hospital. Doctors and nurses pressed by the heavy demands of the more acutely ill patients are sometimes prone to neglect those for whom they know they can do little. Patients are often only too aware of the neglect and the implication of such neglect. As one patient put it, "My doctor does not come to see me any more. He hurries by my room; he does not speak to me; he just waves at me."

How much a little attention can mean to a patient is illustrated by the story of a young woman of 23 who was readmitted to the hospital in the terminal stages of cancer. The patient was aware of the gravity of her condition and, though fearing that death was near, was afraid to admit her fears and never mentioned them. In the course of one of her conversations with the social worker, she mentioned her embarrassment at the constant staining of her nightclothes from draining lesions. Arrangements were made for her to have special gauze pads, whereupon she commented that "the hospital going to all the trouble of providing these special pads makes me feel it isn't all over."

The fact that the social worker accepted without denial all the implications of this remark enabled the patient to express her fears in other ways. At a later date, she commented that the doctors were not paying much attention to her any more—"I guess they gave me up"—following this remark with the plea that the worker continue to come to see her frequently.

It was quite evident that since medical science was helpless, the social worker was unable to make any change in the situation. Nevertheless, these visits had value to the patient in that they made her feel that as long as the social worker came to visit, she still was of some account.

The reaction of this patient illustrates that the service which we can render and which indicates to the patient that he still is worth someone's attention and concern and that "it isn't all over" need not necessarily be spectacular. Such simple services as providing dentures for an elderly woman whose prognosis is poor helps to demonstrate to her better than any spoken reassurance can that she is still considered "worth bothering with" and has a right to be made as comfortable as is possible within our power.

A case comes to mind of a 16-year-old boy suffering from malignant hypertension which caused a rapid progressive destruction of the blood vessels. The doctor did not give him much more than a year to live.

The boy seemed little concerned about being in the hospital. He had had several hospitalizations, was familiar with hospital routine, and accustomed to separation from family and friends. Not subjected to intense physical distress, unaware of the seriousness of his condition, he seemed not at all disturbed by it. What troubled him most was the fact that he was falling behind in his studies and that when he would be ready to return to school, his friends would have outdistanced him.

In view of the reality of the situation and the knowledge that this boy would never return to school, it would have been easy to side-step his concern. Why "waste" the effort and the time involved when we knew that in all probability he would never leave the hospital? It was recognized, however, that giving this boy an opportunity to continue with his studies was not just wasted effort. It meant that we acknowledged his right to do the things he wanted to do and to have desires and plans for the future. Arrangements for bedside instruction were made. The boy was given the opportunity and the satisfaction of doing what he wanted to do as long as he was able to do it, and in this way his rights as a living human being were preserved to the last.

It is true that no matter what we do, we cannot allay the fear and anxiety of the patient who feels that he is failing rapidly or who senses that death is imminent. We can help, however, if our attitude toward such a patient is not, "What can I do for this patient who is going to die within six weeks?" but, "What can I do for this patient who has six weeks to *live?* How can I make these six weeks more comfortable, more satisfying to him?"

THE INCAPACITATED PERSON
IN THE COMMUNITY

The downward trend of an illness and the threat of impending death, representing as they do the ultimate in hopelessness, are not the only situations in which it is as important as it is difficult to preserve the patient's rights as a functioning human being. There are occasions when the need to continue living presents its own serious difficulties, as, for instance, when the patient has to leave the hospital and return home in the face of negligible physical gains. The patient with prolonged illness, unlike his acutely ill counterpart, does not leave his illness behind the closed hospital doors. All too often, prolonged or even permanent disability, complete or partial, is a frequent concomitant and the threat of recurrence is an ever present possibility. Having looked forward to leaving the hospital and resuming his place in the community, the patient may, at the time of discharge, be forced to realize that the possibility of his hopes being fulfilled is slim, or even totally nonexistent.

For the patient discharged with a residual handicap, the seriousness of the problem he will have to face upon his return home and the degree to which his mode of living will be affected, is determined by the extent of his disablity and the amount of readjustment it imposes. Whatever the extent of readjustment required, the very fact that he is no longer in the hospital and yet is unable to function normally in the community brings him face to face with a number of problems. Removal of medical attention without perceptible alteration in his physical condition implies that medical science "has given up," that there is little hope for further improvement or for any change for the better. In view of this, he can no longer consider the situation as temporary and has to acknowledge the permanency of the curtailment of work capacity with all that such a change implies so far as economic security, standard of living of his family, and, consequently, his status in the group, are concerned.

Nor is this all. Under such circumstances, the patient has an additional problem to face, for he has to come to terms with his feelings about himself as an individual and a member of the community in which he lives. Whereas the hospitalized patient is by social sanction absolved from meeting his usual obligations, once he returns home he is constantly reminded of the fact that he is not performing in the way society expects of him or in the way he expects of himself.

If we are to preserve the patient's rights as an individual in the home as well as in the hospital, it is important to remember that in addition to the needs created by his illness, he has the needs common to us all, sick and well. The concept of a full life includes more than a vegetative existence. The patient needs an opportunity for some activity commensurate with his capacity and a sense of not being merely a burden but of being able to contribute to, and share in, the life around him. Deprived of the attention of the medical personnel, the protection of the hospital, and the feeling of security inherent in its routine, the patient must not only look to others in his immediate environment for help with his everyday needs but, even more important, he must look to them for the satisfaction of his emotional needs as well. The attitude of those around him, therefore, becomes the one all-important single factor in assuring for him as satisfying a life as his condition permits.

Such an attitude of understanding and helpfulness is often difficult to maintain. For the patient unable to return to gainful employment or to resume his old place in the world, acutely conscious of his displacement in a setting where he previously had status and authority, the situation is a constant reminder and demonstration of his worthlessness. Unable to change the situation and under pressure of continued frustration, the patient may become unreasonable, faultfinding, and demanding. This coupled with the tyranny which the demands of his physical condition often exercise over other family members is a source of constant aggravation and potential family disharmony.

The understanding of what the situation can mean to the

patient, so important in any attempt to help him, becomes even more difficult to achieve when instead of being confined to the few professional people concerned with his care, such understanding needs to be disseminated among many members of the family and in the community. To counteract this situation, fraught with so much danger for the patient's welfare, advantage can and must be taken of the positive values inherent in long-standing personal relationships and the interest and concern for the patient and his welfare.

In the absence of such interest, the patient's position in the family and the attention he will receive can, nevertheless, be immeasurably enhanced once his feeling of uselessness is minimized. Any contribution the patient can make will help to preserve family harmony, lessen the strain on the patient and on those around him, and increase the chances for peaceful living for all concerned. Even when economic gains are not forthcoming, giving the patient an opportunity to be useful holds the possibility of other values for him and those closely associated with him:

There was, for instance, Mr. U., a 69-year-old widower who was admitted to the hospital with an acute exacerbation of a long-standing stomach ailment.

Mr. U. was never a successful man. Of limited mental capacity, he was never able to do more than unskilled work in the garment industry. His earnings were at all times insufficient for the family's maintenance. His frequent ailments, the forerunners of the chronic condition which brought him to the hospital, further interfered with his working and reduced his earnings.

There was a history of considerable domestic friction. To supplement Mr. U.'s meager earnings, the children were forced to go to work at an early age, foregoing their ambition for further education. They felt deprived and resented their father's inadequacy.

When Mrs. U. died, one of the married daughters took Mr. U. into her home. Mr. U. continued to work sporadically; his financial contribution was slight, hardly covering his own expenses. The daughter kept him out of a sense of duty, but grudgingly. Mr. U.'s share in the life of the family was infinitesimal. He was merely someone she had to put up with, the daughter felt.

While Mr. U. was in the hospital it became evident that he would never be able to return to his former employment. His job, inadequate as it was, had in the past been a means of escaping, at least temporarily, from a home where he felt unwanted. Now even this would be denied him.

In an attempt to provide some activity which could occupy Mr. U.'s time once he was out of the hospital, the occupational therapist was asked to visit Mr. U. He expressed but mild interest in the different projects she suggested and showed no ability in carrying them through. The therapist persevered in her attempts to find something which would engage his interest. One day as she was showing another patient how to make a hooked rug, Mr. U. said he would like to try that.

It soon became evident that here was something that really appealed to him. He had a fine sense of color combinations and was painstaking in his efforts. When Mr. U. was ready to return home, he expressed his desire to continue making hooked rugs, and arrangements were made for him to secure the necessary equipment and supplies.

Seen shortly after his discharge, Mr. U. was busy and happy. His daughter, he said, had asked him whether he would make a rug for her if she would supply the wool. "She is nicer to me than she ever was before." After school, his grandchildren would gather around and watch him, fascinated. Patiently, he would answer their questions as to why he used one color or another. Mr. U. took a great deal of pride in his skill and was eager to exhibit it. Neighbors began to drop in to admire his work, and he volunteered to teach them how to hook rugs. He thought he might be able to sell some and contribute "my share of my upkeep."

For the first time, Mr. U. had a feeling of accomplishment and a sense that he was being looked up to by his family and neighbors.

Difficult and traumatic as the situation may be for the patient who is obviously incapacitated, it is even more difficult for the patient whose illness has few outward manifestations. So much more is expected of him. The protection which hospitalization or visible handicap throws around the patient is removed, and he is left defenseless to cope with the demands made on him. Cognizant of his uselessness, his idleness, and his inability to perform on the usual level, and aware of the stigma attached by society to such idleness, it is no wonder that such a patient feels called upon to explain his inadequacy, and almost to apologize for his existence.

It is obviously impossible to protect the individual patient from the harmful effects of unenlightened community attitudes. The professional team concerned with total medical care has a responsibility, however, to do everything in their power to change these attitudes. This can best be done through a persistent emphasis on an awareness of the patient's desires, needs, and problems extending far beyond the requirements of the disease. Such an attitude, once developed, would replace unproductive pity with a positive respect for the human being regardless of his limitations and a desire to provide a milieu in which he can function and contribute to the utmost of his ability.

It would then be possible to mobilize the community not only to provide the necessary facilities for adequate medical care, but also to provide facilities for enriching the lives of those who, because of their illness, have lost most of the satisfactions they previously enjoyed. Such a change in attitude would make it possible to utilize to the utmost whatever capacities the sick person retains and by so doing increase his feeling of usefulness, worth, and status.

8

REHABILITATION AS PART OF TOTAL MEDICAL CARE

As WE HAVE SEEN, the adjustment which the patient suffering from aftereffects of prolonged illness has to face, once the hospitalization period is over, is a difficult one. Because prolonged illness produces numerous dislocations and affects all areas of living, the patient must become accustomed not only to living with a residual handicap, but also to the way in which this handicap will affect his future work capacity, his social relationships, and his status in the community.

The complete inactivity characteristic of hospital existence and the enforced dependence on others, which illness creates, tend to undermine the dignity of the individual. This becomes particularly apparent when his hospitalization has come to an end and the patient is thrown into the maelstrom of everyday living, where his idleness and helplessness stand out in sharp contrast against the activity around him.

In attempting to preserve his self-respect while adjusting to a new role and way of functioning in his social milieu, the patient may at times be able to rationalize his inability to attain economic independence and even his need to rely on others in matters of self-care. However, living in a culture which emphasizes the importance of self-reliance and of the ability to "earn one's keep," the patient cannot long remain oblivious to his inadequacies. As he encounters repeated frustrations, he becomes acutely aware of the risk of losing his position among his peers, a feeling which is further aggravated by the attitude of others in his environment.

It will be generally agreed that the disabled individual as well as the healthy one is entitled to the inalienable right to the pursuit of happiness, which includes the right to achieve a socially useful and personally satisfying life. If this right is to be preserved, the patient must be helped to achieve fulfillment through the utmost utilization of all his available potentialities, as an active, responsible participant and a functioning member of society.

As we look about us, however, we find ample evidence to indicate that so far as the patient suffering from an irreversible disability is concerned, these basic rights are disregarded only too frequently. Society is too often inclined to regard the disabled individual as being in a somewhat different category, unable to participate in, and contribute to, the community in which he lives. Little if any attention is given to the satisfaction of his inner needs, or to the provision of opportunities for the exercise and development of such capacities as he possesses. It is as if the very fact of his being handicapped is in itself sufficient reason for consigning him to oblivion. And yet, as Dr. Howard A. Rusk, an outstanding proponent of a new approach to the problems of the handicapped, points out, "it is an axiom of rehabilitation that no matter how physically handicapped a man may be, he has far more ability than disability." [1]

Society is slowly coming to the realization that not only does the disabled individual share with his nondisabled neighbor the common aspiration to be self-sustaining, but that the disability does not deprive him of the right to a full, productive, and satisfying life, and that he, as well as his more fortunate able-bodied counterpart, must be given the opportunity to derive the usual satisfactions from his social relationships as an accepted and respected member of his group. Little by little it is being recognized that the disabled person wants to have an interest in life and not merely "kill time";

[1] Rusk, "Recovery in Poland," p. 49.

he wants to be of use so that he may retain his self-respect, and he wants to be wanted and thus be sure that he retains the respect and love of others. Though the disability may make the achievement of these goals difficult, a great deal can be accomplished, given an acceptance of the need to provide means for the restoration of the incapacitated individual, and a willingness to adjust the goals to which such restoration can aspire in each individual case.

We tend to forget that the activities of daily living, so much taken for granted and performed so automatically by the able-bodied, become major undertakings for the disabled, demanding the utmost concentration and strenuous exercise. Even the achievement of such humble tasks as caring for some of his basic personal needs promotes in the individual a feeling of mastery and a sense of belonging, participating, and contributing, even though to a limited extent, in the life around him. This feeling in and of itself serves to comfort, strengthen, and support the individual. It is to him an indication of the end to the helpless existence to which he had been hitherto condemned, and represents the first step in regaining his rightful place in the scheme of things. The process of rehabilitation must therefore begin with the minutiae of everyday living, and the professional personnel concerned with the patient's care, as well as family members, must adopt a new attitude and a changed mode of behavior toward him. As stated by Dr. N. K. Covalt, "doctors, nurses, and relatives need to 'unlearn' waiting upon patients as a form of good medical care, but need to learn methods and the psychology of teaching the patient to care for himself." [2]

This represents a new understanding of what we mean by rehabilitation. Vocational placement is no longer the only goal to which rehabilitation aspires. Its character and scope have been enlarged in line with our greater awareness of the problems presented by our handicapped population and our

[2] Covalt, p. 98.

increased knowledge of the way in which these problems can be met. The responsibility of the medical profession is extended to embrace not only the provision of medical and nursing care, but equally as much the achievement of maximal physical restoration through the utilization of all potentials of which the patient is capable, in such a way that, in spite of his residual handicap, he may derive satisfactions from making whatever contribution he can to communal living. This new approach has broadened the concept of rehabilitation and heightened our appreciation of the goals to which the handicapped individual can aspire, with due recognition of his limitations as well as his capacities. Once such acceptance is assured, it becomes possible for the handicapped person to relate to others on a realistic basis, without an overwhelming feeling of inferiority, without the need to apologize for his existence or to compete on a level which in actuality he cannot attain.

THE CHANGING EMPHASIS IN REHABILITATION

The general concept of the need to rehabilitate the disabled individual is now new. Even before use of the term "rehabilitation" as we now understand it became popular, certain forms of rehabilitation were being practiced as accepted components of medical care.

The physician who through his knowledge and skill brought the patient back to health, or who saw to it that he be provided with an artificial limb following amputation, was actually "rehabilitating" him. The nurse who encouraged and helped the patient to ambulate after a prolonged period in bed participated in restoring him to his former capacity. The social worker who secured a sedentary job for the patient who was no longer able to engage in door-to-door selling, or who made arrangements to move a cardiac patient from his third-floor walk-up apartment, was actively contributing to his rehabilitation. The importance of the emphasis on rehabilitation as we now know it lies in the concept of the person as an integrated human being, in the recognition of the need for organized rehabilitation facilities, and in the purposeful utilization of numerous professional skills to cope with the manifold problems inherent in any attempt to guide the handicapped toward independence.

This change in emphasis did not occur suddenly. It is the result of steady and progressive growth. From the humble beginnings of the first recognition of a need, the concept has developed gradually through the years, as we achieved a greater awareness of the extent and nature of the problems a handicap creates, and recognition of the value of rehabilitation services in dealing with these problems. Today we see an increased understanding of the interrelation of physical, social, and emotional factors in the rehabilitation problems which confront us, and the need to handle all these problems, utilizing a variety of skills in order to arrive at a plan of treatment which meets the patient's needs and one which is likely to bring satisfactory results.

The definition adopted by the National Council on Rehabilitation in 1943 is still valid today. It states that "rehabilitation is restoration of the handicapped to the fullest physical, mental, social, vocational, and economic usefulness of which they are capable." And the Commission on Chronic Illness defines rehabilitation as being "a program designed to enable the individual who is physically disabled, chronically ill, or convalescing, to live and to work to the utmost of his capacity. It is an integral part of clinical, non-institutional, and community responsibility in meeting the problems of chronic illness." [3]

These definitions do not limit rehabilitation to the narrow confines of economic productivity, but see it as being concerned with all the facets of the patient's adjustment. The aim of rehabilitation is no longer seen as solely preparation

[3] "Rehabilitation, a Hospital-Community Challenge," p. 2.

for the resumption of former duties and responsibilities. In fact, no limits are set to the goals toward which rehabilitation may strive, except in so far as it acknowledges the limits existing within each individual's capacities. While for one patient the ultimate goal may be a return to full independent functioning, for another it may be but the development of his capacity to leave the confines of the hospital, or it may be any of the intermediate stages between these two extremes.

As is true of all other forms of welfare activity, efforts at rehabilitating the handicapped were first undertaken by private charitable organizations thoroughly familiar with the serious and extensive sequelae of physical disability. It was soon recognized that such ameliorative measures, though important in themselves, were inadequate to solve a problem so vast in its implications, since these measures reached but a small group of those afflicted; even for this small group the results achieved often failed to return the disabled to some measure of self-sufficiency.

The term "rehabilitation" as we now understand it was first introduced during the First World War by military hospitals to designate those techniques which helped to reduce the incapacity of military personnel and to return men to active duty. The success these techniques frequently achieved led to the conviction that they could be fruitfully utilized in peacetime. This, in turn, led to the establishment of rehabilitation services for veterans who had returned to civilian life. The first steps toward making legal provision of similar benefits for civilians were taken during the Second World War when the nation needed to utilize its manpower to the utmost in an all-out effort to maintain and expand defense industries.

More and more, within recent years, efforts at rehabilitating the handicapped have become associated with the enactment of federal legislation.

The first rehabilitation act was passed in 1920 in response to public concern for the disabled veterans of World War I.

Known as the National Rehabilitation Act (Public Law 36) it provided for grants to states for vocational training, counseling, and job placement of veterans and was administered by the Federal Board of Vocational Education. Among the numerous expansions and modifications which followed was Public Law 113 (Bardon–La Follette bill) which provided for the rehabilitation of disabled civilians with special emphasis on the rehabilitation of injured workers. The federal support resulted in substantial progress, and rehabilitation took its place as one of the important factors in the treatment of all handicapped and disabled persons. With increased experience, the concept of what constitutes adequate rehabilitation services was broadened both so far as the facilities provided and the clientele served, and measures were taken to insure the functioning of the program on a more efficient, stable, and permanent basis. While the primary impetus was supplied by the need to man the nation's defense industries, it had, nevertheless, the effect of drawing attention to the human values involved. Nowadays, we are inclined to regard rehabilitation as an integral part of the activities of the federal government in its over-all concern with the health and welfare of the people.

We now see the Federal Vocational Rehabilitation program providing services for school dropouts, rejected draftees, the disabled poor, the blind, the deaf, the mentally retarded, victims of heart disease, cancer, and stroke as well as the aged. In addition, the 1954 amendments provided authority for a program of support for training in several disciplines in colleges, universities, and other institutions.[4] All this does not negate the fact that "whatever changes were contemplated in the legislation, the aim of the public program remained the same: enhancement of the personal dignity of disabled people through the ability to perform useful work."[5]

Important as are the activities of the federal government,

[4] Vocational Rehabilitation Administration, p. 376.   [5] Ibid., p. 369.

they nonetheless fail to meet the total needs of the disabled among us, for their emphasis is on economic productivity and is geared toward getting the disabled person back to work. In line with this expressed objective, eligibility requirements, as outlined in the law, emphasize potential employability. The law expressly provides that the individual must be of working age, that his disability must constitute an employment handicap which, as a result of the rehabilitation efforts, will be sufficiently improved to enable him to engage in remunerative work. The annual reports of the Office of Vocational Rehabilitation of the Federal Security Agency emphasize the economic values of the program as a reason for its further development and expansion, and the statistics presented draw attention to the number of persons returned to gainful employment, the amount of their earnings, and point to the fact that through rehabilitation these people not only have been made independent, but have actually returned to the government in taxes more than the amount spent on their training. Thus the various legislative acts, as well as the pronouncements of authorities in charge of rehabilitation facilities, both private and public, amply demonstrate the fact that in the past emphasis was put on economic gains, and rehabilitation was conceived as being primarily the return to industrial productivity.

Recent developments bear witness to an increased appreciation of the fact that for some patients physical medicine alone may not be sufficient to insure total rehabilitation and the successful assumption of full responsibility for independent functioning in the community upon discharge from a hospital. A somewhat new approach to rehabilitation is the basis of the program being conducted at the Restoration Center at the Veterans Administration Hospital in East Orange, New Jersey.

The Center, having completed construction and staffing, began operating in June, 1964, with the intent to explore and develop an approach to total rehabilitation, termed "res-toration." The Center is under the direction of Dr. James C. Hart with a staff including an assistant director who is a physician, nurses, social workers, psychologists, physical medi-cine therapists, dieticians, as well as a director of program research and evaluation. It aims to "close or bridge the gap between hospitalization and return to non-hospital indepen-dence in the community viewed in its broadest sense." The closing of the gap is intended to break the pattern of cyclic readmissions as well as to reduce the undesirable necessity to devote acute hospital facilities for the extended time neces-sary for the formulation of a stable and appropriate discharge plan.

The Restoration Center approach is based upon the inter-relation between staff, physical facility, administrative and program principles, time element, the community, and the veteran, each one of these being utilized as a defined thera-peutic tool leading to the desired goal of total restoration. Veterans are referred to the Restoration Center by the hospital physician when it is determined by him that con-tinued hospitalization is no longer necessary. The final deci-sion to accept or reject the veteran for the restoration program is determined by the Center staff based on their evaluation of the veteran's need for the services which the program has to offer, as well as a reasonable expectation of his eventual improvement and ability to function in the com-munity. Neither diagnosis nor age are determining factors in establishing eligibility for admission. To be chosen for the program, the veteran must have reached a point in his medical treatment where he no longer requires hospitaliza-tion, is capable of caring for his personal needs with minimal assistance, can participate in the required activities of the Center, and can follow the prescribed medical regimen.

This residential facility consists of four interconnected single-story buildings—colorful, cheerful, geared to the needs of the program with a deliberate effort to duplicate conditions which the veteran would be likely to encounter in the community. From both a prosthetic and a therapeutic viewpoint, careful attention is paid to the veteran's reaction to these surroundings and to such difficulties as he may encounter in adjusting to them.

The veteran is admitted to the program for a period of one year, if necessary, to give sufficient time for evaluation, treatment, trial periods of adjustment to gradually increased responsibility, and for adequate discharge planning. The time limit can be used effectively by the staff to motivate the unmotivated veteran as well as to provide for the deliberate use of "timing" in the development of the rehabilitative discharge plan. Trial visits, leaves of absence, and passes are utilized liberally as a part of the therapeutic program and follow-up evaluation. The adjacent hospital provides specialty consultative services as well as temporary hospitalization, as the need arises, for emergency care or for elective treatment deemed necessary for the fulfillment of the eventual rehabilitative goal.

As a basic part of their gradual assumption of responsibility, the veterans are required to be independently mobile in the Center. They go to the cafeteria, for instance, where they carry their own trays. They are taught to select such foods as their diet requires. As a part of the self-administered medication program, they are expected to go to the pharmacy, located in the main hospital building to have their prescriptions filled. Learning to use simple kitchen and laundry equipment is part of the routine of self-care for those who intend to live alone.

The community is dynamically involved, utilizing individuals, groups, business establishments, and social agencies in the exploration of vocational potential, training, and placement; in securing adequate living arrangements, and in developing activities designed to meet social and recreational needs. Contact with the community to secure such help as the veteran might need is undertaken well in advance of the discharge.

The veteran himself is expected to become involved with the staff in his own rehabilitative program in decision-making, in assuming responsibility for his progress and for increased independent functioning, a concept which is in direct contrast to the traditionally passive role required of the hospital patient.

Five hundred and ninety-three veterans were admitted to the Center within the first two years of its existence, and the Center functioned at capacity within the first twelve months. Applications were received from 17 states, other than New Jersey, and the District of Columbia. Geographic spread, in the development phase, has included Texas, Florida, and New Hampshire. The veterans, ranging in age from 19 to 93, came from general medical as well as psychiatric hospitals; almost half had neurological or psychiatric disabilities.

By June 30, 1966, the end of the second year, 196 veterans had been discharged as restored to maximal capacity. Initial follow-up indicates that there has been a satisfactory adjustment to community life in from 75 percent to 90 percent of the cases, depending upon the length of time in the Center and the discharge goal. It is of importance to note that a significant number of these patients had particularly difficult and complex problems, manifesting behavior not easily tolerated by the community, as well as extremely long periods of hospitalization prior to admission to the Restoration Center, in some cases as long as 18 consecutive years.

It is felt that this kind of total rehabilitation—restoration to community living, varying from the complete dependence characteristic of hospital living to a semiprotective, supportive environment before being exposed to independent community living—is of positive advantage to the patients, the hospital, and the community. Accordingly, with the increased awareness of the need for a dynamic approach to chronic illness and the need for extended rehabilitation efforts, similar facilities are proposed elsewhere in the United States to provide the needed geographic distribution of the services.

THE MEANING OF REHABILITATION AS IT APPLIES TO THE PERMANENTLY DISABLED

Even though various social and personal values accruing as a result of rehabilitation are recognized, and despite the progress made within recent years in broadening the concept of rehabilitation, we have as yet paid but scant attention to those who cannot hope to return to full working capacity, but who nevertheless need to regain some measure of self-reliance.

What does rehabilitation mean to the individual with a residual incapacity who therefore cannot aspire to eventual economic independence? What can be done to help him achieve a sense of worthwhile living by increasing his ability to be self-reliant? What substitute satisfactions can be provided for him to compensate for loss of status in the workaday world?

As we review the situation, it becomes abundantly clear that for the patient for whom eventual employability is an unattainable goal, but who has the capacity to achieve a degree of self-care, facilities to enable him to do so are still lacking. If we subscribe to the doctrine that a severely impaired individual has a right to happiness and participation in normal living in so far as his condition permits, then the responsibility for the provision of such facilities becomes a must as the next step in our social planning for him. The importance of such a step assumes added significance when we consider the ever increasing number of people in the age groups in which illnesses of prolonged duration are likely to prevail, leaving their victims with an incapacitating residual impairment.

As was previously mentioned, the National Health Survey found that there were about 22.2 million persons with one or more chronic disabling conditions involving activity limitation. The Vocational Rehabilitation Administration estimates that some 3.7 million of these would be eligible and could profit from their services. Of these, a "total of 134,859 mentally or physically disabled persons [were] rehabilitated to useful work" during 1965.[6] These figures emphasize the vastness of the problem with which we are dealing, particularly when we remember that the numbers quoted apply only to those individuals who have an employment handicap, and do not include those handicapped persons who are ineligible for the services of the Vocational Rehabilitation Administration. Other authorities are in substantial agreement.

In attempting to decide how many of the people afflicted with such incapacitating residues of prolonged illness can aspire to even partial economic independence, we must again rely on estimates, since no definite figures are available. According to Shortley, one fourth of those disabled could probably never function in industry.[7] And Dr. Henry H. Kessler, on the basis of long experience with problems of rehabilitation, estimates that about 40 percent could be "partially productive if their disabilities are considered and they are placed in employment where physical demands do not exceed capacities." [8]

It is self-evident that extensive rehabilitation facilities are not always necessary to help severely handicapped individuals, a number of them being able to function without such help. Mr. Young, for instance, who had lost both lower extremities, was able to continue at his trade as watchmaker. Because he had always operated his business from his home, transportation difficulties were obviated, and although he

---

[6] Vocational Rehabilitation Administration (formerly Office of Vocational Rehabilitation), Annual Report 1965, p. 369.
[7] Shortley, p. 264.   [8] Kessler, p. 88.

had to adjust to his physical condition, he was not faced with an employment handicap.

Important as are the values inherent in vocational rehabilitation with its goal of complete or even partial financial independence, we must recognize that in the past the very emphasis on *vocational* rehabilitation has tended to obscure the simple truth that there is a group of handicapped people whose disabilities cannot be overcome by existing medical knowledge and for whom a vocational goal is unattainable, but who, given the necessary help, can learn to function in their daily living with considerable satisfaction to themselves and to those close to them.

To those of us whose primary interest is the preservation and enhancement of human dignity and securing as satisfactory a life as possible for the severely afflicted, it is important that a rehabilitation program have as its aim the maximal utilization of the individual's capacities, the development of self-reliance and independence despite existing disabilities, even though the goal may be less than complete restoration.

Recognizing the fact that rehabilitation services can be provided on different levels, it becomes our responsibility to determine what services are required in each individual instance. This means that for each patient we must know the extent of his handicap, what he knows about it, what his previous attainments were, and the degree to which his disability interferes with the resumption of his previous way of life. Equally important is an understanding of the patient's feelings about his disability, how he uses it, what satisfactions it provides, what frustrations it causes, and his willingness to accommodate himself to a new way of functioning.

While we may speak of the maximal goal of rehabilitation as being the attainment of optimal satisfaction of the desires of the physically or emotionally handicapped person, his family, and the community, it is not easy to determine either the maximal or the minimal goals to which we may aspire in any individual case. It may mean, on the one end of the scale, a return to full economic productivity, and on the other, merely the development of the ability to indulge in simple recreational or avocational activities that have no economic value, but are of considerable value psychologically and socially. For one patient rehabilitation may mean merely being able to take care of all or part of his physical needs in bed; for another, it may be attaining the ability to get out of bed, to use a wheel chair, crutches, or canes, to learn to walk. This too is rehabilitation. Regardless of the degree of self-reliance finally achieved, given the proper motivation the handicapped person can perform on a level which approaches the limits of his capacities, and can derive satisfaction from being useful even though the usefulness is in terms other than that of economic return.

Among the disabled, those whose problems of adjustment have until now received the least attention are the handicapped housewives. In this neglect we see the end result of the hitherto prevalent emphasis on economic returns from rehabilitation efforts; for a rehabilitation program for the disabled housewife promises no such rewards. In view of our society's attitude as it relates to the importance of the home and the family, it is essential that greater emphasis be placed on making it possible for the disabled housewife to resume and maintain her role in the family circle.

It is encouraging to note that we have been moving steadily to a broader interpretation of the aims of rehabilitation to include other than potential breadwinners, with particular emphasis on the needs of the disabled woman, a concentration on improvements in job methods, the adjustment of the physical facilities in the home to her requirements, and the manufacture of many devices to enable her to perform her usual duties. Some of these devices show considerable ingenuity in the adaptation of everyday utensils;

the production of others requires a certain amount of engineering knowledge. It is gratifying to see that an increasing number of commercial firms are willing not only to undertake the manufacture of special home appliances for the handicapped housewife, but to make such adjustments as may be necessary to meet individual needs.

How important attention to the problems of the disabled homemaker can be is clearly illustrated in the case of Mrs. Ross:

At the time Mrs. Ross was stricken with rheumatoid arthritis, she was earning a living by doing embroidery. Little by little, as her illness progressed, she was forced to abandon this fine work and was reduced to a less skillful occupation with a consequent reduction in her earning capacity.

Finally, at the age of 50 she had to give up work altogether and was forced to make her home with a married daughter. To maintain some vestige of her independence, and the feeling that she was not utterly useless, she undertook part of the household responsibilities. Her crippled condition made housework slow and laborious, but she persisted in it until the arthritic process in her toes forced her into complete immobility. The necessity of becoming a burden on her daughter without being able to give anything in return made Mrs. Ross miserable and depressed.

It was quite evident that rehabilitation in the usual sense was impracticable, and the primary concern was to help this woman to minimize her dependency and thus dispel the discouragement and depression which threatened to engulf her.

After all possible medical treatment was completed, Mrs. Ross was provided with a pair of special shoes; kitchen equipment was rearranged, and a special wheel chair enabled her to move around more comfortably. Slowly she was able to resume those household duties which she had previously performed.

The amount of rehabilitation possible in this particular instance was admittedly minimal. However, within the limits of the irremediable physical handicap, the maximum that could be expected for this patient was achieved by returning to her some measure of independence and the feeling of being a contributing member of the family group.

It is self-evident that this newer concept of what constitutes adequate rehabilitation services involves so many aspects of the patient's life that no one professional discipline is equipped to handle them all. Any attack on a problem so all-encompassing and so pervasive in its implications, if it is to serve the common goal of maximal benefit to the patient, requires the combined efforts of numerous professional skills, which must be so coordinated and integrated as to obtain a rounded view of the problem and make possible an effective way of working together.

This concept of different professions working together in a teamwork relationship has become widely accepted. It has captured the imagination of the helping professions and has proved to be a valuable, often an essential tool.

What is teamwork?

According to the dictionary definition, teamwork is "work done by a number of associates, usually each doing a clearly defined portion, but all subordinating personal prominence to the efficiency of the whole." A more detailed definition, outlining the goals as well as the methods of teamwork, has been advanced:

Teamwork as it applies to the total rehabilitation center is a close, cooperative, democratic, multiprofessional union devoted to a common purpose—the best treatment of the fundamental need of the individual. Its members work through a combined and integrated diagnosis; flexible, dynamic planning; proper timing and sequence of treatment, and balance in action. It is an organismic group distinct in its parts, yet acting as a unit, i.e., no important action is taken by members of one profession without the consent of the group. Just as the individual acts as an interrelated whole, and not as a sum of his characteristics, so must the profession act, think, interpret, and contribute toward a diagnosis which is the product of all, and a treatment plan which is dynamic to accommodate the changes which a dynamic human organism is constantly making.[9]

This definition implies the recognition on the part of all participants that there exists a problem requiring attention, a desire to solve it by active participation, a recognition by each member of his inability to solve it singlehanded, a clear understanding of one's own function, an appreciation of, and respect for, the function of the other team members and the contribution they can make, a flexibility in adjusting one's own part in the process, a willingness to share in the helping process on a give-and-take basis and to arrive at a common solution with the primary goal of the patient's welfare as the focus of activity.

The multiphasic study which is the concern of the team approach, as it functions in modern rehabilitation projects, deals with an evaluation of the patient's ability as it is affected by his medical condition and the limitations it imposes, his personality make-up, vocational aspirations, and social and emotional needs. The contribution of each team member, made on the basis of a particular, highly developed skill, must identify the need as it appears in his specific area, determine the limits within which he can function in the patient's best interests, and interpret his understanding to the other team members. In view of the complexity of the problem, such a division of responsibility appears to be unavoidable in our age of specialization. It has been found through experience that whatever disadvantages are inherent in what appears to be a fragmented approach are outweighed by the advantages which accrue from the intensive study of each particular aspect of the situation, and from the need to interpret one's point of view to other professional personnel, enabling, as it does, each member to get away from the

[9] Whitehouse, p. 46.

narrow, one-dimensional characteristics of his own specialty. The type of collaboration implied demands a high level of professional maturity and results in better integrated treatment and a more effective rehabilitation program.

Because of the multiplicity of functions represented on the team, it is essential to clarify the specialized skills which its members bring to the solution of the patient's problem, since they all must make their contributions purposefully focused and related to their particular line of activity. No definite statement can be made as to how many professions should be represented on a rehabilitation team. It may include physicians, nurses, social workers, psychiatrists, psychologists, physical therapists, occupational therapists, vocational counselors, and many others, or any combination of these, depending upon the auspices under which the team functions, and the type of problem it is called upon to consider. Nor need all the professional skills necessarily be represented in every instance. The effectiveness of the team depends not so much on the variety of professions represented, but rather on whether these professions are the ones which can contribute most effectively to the understanding of the particular problem and to its solution. Most of all, the effectiveness of the team will depend on whether there exists an atmosphere of mutual respect and understanding, so that each participant can express and interpret his point of view freely while at the same time maintaining the necessary respect for the contribution of others.

In discussing the contributions of the different professional disciplines, an attempt will be made to point out not only those aspects which are unique to that specialty, but also those which are equally applicable to others in the professional team.

THE ROLE OF THE PHYSICIAN

Since our discussion concerns physically disabled individuals, the determination of the patient's medical status and the type and amount of physical exertion he can undertake is at the core of all rehabilitation efforts. While it is true that medical advances have made it possible in some instances to attack disability at its source, preventing its crippling effects, or lessening the amount of residual handicap, nevertheless many other conditions still leave their victims with some degree of impairment. When this is the case, even the most effective medical care represents but the beginning of the physician's role in the process of restoring the patient to such economic and social usefulness as his residual handicap permits. Our present philosophy reaffirms the conviction that "it has always been inherent in the tradition of medicine that the doctor's work does not cease with the mere cure of his patient's disease or the correction of his disability, but only when he has done his utmost to enable the patient to function again as an active member of the community." [10] This philosophy applies equally to all types of illness and disability regardless of the degree of severity.

Nor are the physician's recommendations as to desirable rehabilitation plans a once-for-all decision. Rehabilitation being a dynamic process and the patient's condition being subject to change, plans must often be altered in view of the patient's reaction to them. Therefore, if maximal rehabilitation is to be achieved, periodic medical reevaluations are important to the team members as well as to the patient. The team members look to the physician not only for a constant reappraisal of the patient's disabilities and limitations but, even more important, for an evaluation of the remaining strengths possessed by the patient which point the direction for future rehabilitation planning.

So far as the patient is concerned, the physician's interest in his welfare, as evidenced by periodic examinations and discussion of potentials for useful living, helps to build the pa-

[10] Fishbein, p. 1.

tient's confidence in himself and to provide the reassurance necessary to alleviate such fears and anxieties as arise when he is confronted with tasks of increasing difficulty.

THE PSYCHIATRIST'S DOUBLE ROLE

As a member of the rehabilitation team, the psychiatrist fulfills a double role by being available to provide direct help to the patient, when necessary, as well as consultation to the other team members with such difficulties as may arise during the rehabilitation process. So far as the patient is concerned, the psychiatrist carries the responsibility for diagnosis and treatment of the patient's emotional reactions just as the physician has the primary responsibility for the diagnosis and treatment of the physical condition.

Because of their varying personality structures and diverse emotional needs, patients react differently not only to the disability itself but also to the efforts taken to overcome it. For example, the patient's attitude of invalidism and dependency, developed over a long period of enforced inactivity, as well as his fear of relapse may result in a reluctance to undertake any type of work. Or the patient may react with depression to the slowness of the progress, interpreting it as an indication of the hopelessness of his condition. The patient's reactions may vary not only in relation to the program as a whole, but also in relation to the different stages of the process, and he may need help in overcoming his reluctance to take the next step toward achieving greater self-reliance, help which the psychiatrist is eminently equipped to give. How important these emotional problems can be, has been brought out in a survey in one rehabilitation center. It was found that "50% of all patients had real emotional problems, which if left unsolved, would have completely negated the physical rehabilitation program." [11]

While helping the patient, the psychiatrist can also help

[11] Rusk, "Lack of Trained Personnel Felt in Rehabilitation Field," p. 46.

the team members by contributing his understanding of the patient's changing reactions, and the way in which the various steps in the rehabilitation process may either meet the patient's needs or threaten his emotional balance. Given such help, the rehabilitation team can then have a better grasp of the dynamics of the patient's acceptance, rejection, or rebellion in the face of proposed plans, as well as of the amount of strain, frustration, or setback he can endure. This increased understanding can then be translated into action, and the goals of the program can be adjusted to meet the patient's emotional as well as his physical needs.

THE FUNCTION OF THE NURSE

The care of the sick has, through the years, involved the nurse, as a vital member of the health team, in a close working relationship with the physician in their joint efforts to prolong life and alleviate suffering. This role has evolved, keeping pace with the altered concept of what constitutes adequate medical care. In line with such changes, the nurse nowadays is not only concerned with the physical care required by the patient, but sees the patient's disability as affecting numerous facets of his life and his plans for the future.

The increase in health services, the expansion of medical knowledge, and the changes in medical practice impose upon the nurse the ever increasing responsibility for absorbing the new knowledge and its implications if she is to collaborate on a professional level with the medical staff and others who deal with the patient. The complexities of the modern medical institution, however, have brought the nurse more and more into clinic management, coordination of services, and the supervision of nonprofessional personnel, thus restricting her availability for the actual care of the sick.

The concern about the nature of available nursing care led to recognition of the need to study priorities in the nursing function and the changes that might ensue. This recognition found expression in a statement recently issued by the American Nurses' Association, outlining the scope of nursing practice, defining the different functions involved in nursing care, and recommending the educational preparation required for the discharge of these functions. This statement expresses the view of the leadership of the profession with emphasis on the fact that "education for those who work in nursing should take place in institutions of higher learning within the general system of education." [12]

The process of rendering nursing care is seen as involving two areas of function, namely, professional nursing practice and technical nursing practice with assistance from persons in "health service occupations" available to these two groups.

The professional nurse is seen as the person with primary responsibility for care of the patient, for helping the patient and his family understand the patient's illness and the preventive measures essential to safeguard his health. In addition, she has the responsibility for collaborating with those in other disciplines and "transmitting the ever-expanding body of knowledge in nursing to those within the profession and outside of it." The "minimum preparation for beginning professional nursing practice at the present time should be a baccalaureate degree."

The technical nurse has highly skilled knowledge and understanding of a variety of complex machines essential for the treatment of the patient and would be able to evaluate "the patient's immediate physical and emotional reactions to therapy and take measures to alleviate distress." She knows "when to act and when to seek more expert guidance."

Working with and under the supervision of the professional nurse, the technical nurse would be an integral part of the team, participating with others in the planning of the ongoing care of the patient. An "associate degree education in

[12] Position Paper on Education for Nursing, pp. 106–11.

nursing" is considered a prerequisite to enable her to discharge this role.

The variety of responsibilities required of professional and technical nurses indicate the need of other personnel, such as nurses' aides, orderlies, and others, to perform delegated tasks and thus free the nurses for their primary responisbilities. It is recommended that such assistants receive short, intensive preservice training in vocational education institutions, this training to be supplemented by in-service orientation and on-the-job training for the specific tasks assigned to them.

While the Position Paper is concerned primarily with the educational requirements for the changing roles of the nurse, its implications for the nurse who functions as a member of the rehabilitation team are self-evident. The nurse who ministers to the patient's medical needs has an unequaled opportunity to observe his reactions and his feelings about himself and his illness. As the nurse learns to pay increased attention to the patient's emotional as well as to his physical well-being, as she learns to listen to what lies behind the spoken word, she can collaborate more effectively with others in making such plans as would be most beneficial to the patient's total welfare.

The following two instances are illustrative of collaborative efforts between the nurse and the social worker, leading to better patient care. The first shows how the nurse's observations and knowledge can be helpful in planning:

Mr. N. came to the attention of the social worker when he was ready for discharge and the doctors found that discharge plans repeatedly bogged down. It appeared to the doctors that Mr. N.'s wife did not want her husband to come home. Before making further plans, the social worker spoke to the nurse who knew Mrs. N., having seen her on many occasions during her husband's hospital stay. The nurse described Mrs. N. as a considerate, thoughtful person who was genuinely concerned about her husband's illness. It was the nurse's opinion that Mrs. N. must have a good reason for refusing to take her husband home.

The nurse's evaluation of Mrs. N.'s character inevitably influenced the social worker's approach to the problem. She learned from Mrs. N. that her resistance to her husband's return sprang from the fact that she was laboring under very real difficulties. Aware of her husband's medical condition, she realized that he would not be receiving the care he needed if he returned home, since she had to continue working to provide for the family.

Alternate plans were discussed and Mrs. N. and the social worker together made arrangements for nursing home care until such time as Mr. N. could assume more responsibility for meeting his everyday needs.[13]

Similarly, the social worker's knowledge of a situation can help provide better care for the patient and eliminate the barriers of prejudice and judgmental attitudes. The following can serve as an illustration:

Mr. A. proved to be a source of constant irritation to the nursing staff. He demanded constant attention, way beyond the nurses' ability to provide. He used the nurses' time to talk about his past successes, spoke about his high earning capacity prior to hospitalization, and the important part he played in community affairs. Unable to admit that a private room was beyond his means, he maintained that the only reason he was on the ward was because he wanted to be assured of the interest of the chief of the medical service. This behavior was naturally irritating to the nurses, who considered him a "braggart." In so far as it was possible, they tried to avoid him.

The social worker, aware of Mr. A.'s situation, was able to explain his behavior on the basis of loss of status which his inability to continue as the breadwinner represented to him, and consequently his need to impress others by continual references to his previous achievements. As the nurses understood the basis

[13] Field, "The Nurse and the Social Worker on the Hospital Team," p. 695.

of his "bragging" and his insatiable need for attention, they were able to ignore the first and to give him an increased amount of attention. Gradually, the patient's demands decreased. This, in turn, meant less irritation on the part of the nurses and consequently better nursing care. The vicious circle was broken.[14]

THE ROLE OF THE OCCUPATIONAL THERAPIST

Occupational therapy has been defined as "any activity, mental or physical, medically prescribed and professionally guided to aid a patient in recovery from disease or injury." [15] It has been widely accepted as an integral part of hospital treatment and is now recognized as being not merely diversional in character, but as having an important place in the scheme of comprehensive medical care. The training "involves the physical re-conditioning of the patient through a carefully devised exercise and activity program in order to make him able to handle his body in the most efficient way so that he will be as independent as possible." [16]

Not only are these physical accomplishments important in themselves, by augmenting the patient's ability to participate in activities of daily living, but they also have a great psychological value. As the patient demonstrates to himself that, despite his handicap, there are areas in which he can be proficient, he acquires a new sense of achievement, security, and freedom from dependence on others in matters of self-care. It is a source of strength on which the patient can draw as he is called upon to meet one challenge after another.

In the course of her work, the occupational therapist, like other members of the team, has the opportunity to observe the patient. Because of her specialized concern, these observations will center on the patient's work interest, his powers of concentration, his attention span, all of which have a bearing in gearing future activities and on the ultimate goals to be set in planning a rehabilitation program.

[14] *Ibid.*, p. 695.   [15] McNary, p. 10.   [16] Buchwald, p. 3.

THE PHYSICAL THERAPIST AND HIS CONTRIBUTION

Physical therapy has been defined as the "treatment of disease or injury by means of heat, cold, light, scientific massage, therapeutic exercise, water and electricity." [17] Whether the goal is complete self-maintenance or minimal self-care, physical therapy helps in the process of recovery to the limit imposed by the patient's physical condition, either through prevention of deterioration, which so often accompanies disuse, or by active restoration.

Its value has been demonstrated since 1919, and it is generally agreed that some form of physical therapy can be administered throughout the patient's stay in the hospital, provided his physical condition is such that in the opinion of the physician he can make constructive use of it. Physical therapy is considered to be an indispensable tool in overcoming the inactivity necessitated by illness and an enforced stay in bed. In common with occupational therapy, it helps enhance the patient's sense of achievement, and its results can be measured not only by increased physical ability, but by the courage and sense of security the patient attains.

The physical therapist brings to the rehabilitation team a specialized knowledge of muscle action, and his function extends into areas of prevention, treatment, and retraining. This professional contribution can help the team to delimit what can be expected of the patient in so far as his physical functioning is concerned.

THE ROLE OF THE PSYCHOLOGIST

The degree of return to normal or near normal functioning which the patient can attain is conditioned not only by his physical and emotional state, but also by his level of intelligence. The determination of the intelligence level and of the individual's aptitudes becomes the responsibility of the

[17] Elson, p. 3.

psychologist, and represents his specialized contribution to the team by helping to determine the type of occupation the patient can pursue. In addition to conducting psychometric testing the psychologist has an opportunity to secure a considerable amount of information and understanding regarding the patient's emotional make-up. To be of maximum usefulness this information must be supplemented by the psychologist's observations of the patient's reactions, which, coordinated with the observations of the other team members, provide useful guides for future planning.

THE CONTRIBUTION OF THE VOCATIONAL COUNSELOR

The contribution of the vocational counselor becomes of primary importance when actual occupational placement is being considered as a goal possible of achievement. By becoming acquainted with a patient's past work history, interests, and skills, the counselor can determine the degree to which a particular line of activity will most nearly meet that patient's intellectual and economic needs. Such an appraisal, including the patient's wishes and hopes for the future, is essential whether the patient is apparently able to consider a return to his former occupation, whether some minor modification of the conditions of his employment is necessary, or whether he requires training for another line of work.

All the information thus secured must be evaluated in the light of the counselor's specialized skills and of his knowledge of community resources. Nor is the determination of vocational goals the only service rendered by the vocational counselor. Having helped the patient in the selection of, and preparation for, a particular occupation, it becomes the vocational counselor's responsibility to make a careful interpretation to the employer of the assets the patient possesses, as a means of overcoming any unfavorable reaction to his physical limitations. In addition, through continued interest in the patient's progress the counselor helps to smooth over difficulties as they arise in the course of employment, thus preventing discouragement and setbacks.

Essentially, the services which the vocational counselor provides for the handicapped are the same as those provided for the able-bodied. However, these services must be more specialized, as well as more extensive and intensive.

THE SOCIAL WORKER AS PART OF
THE REHABILITATION TEAM

Throughout the preceding pages there are numerous indications of the role of the social worker in helping patients deal with the various problems with which illness confronts them. Here, our primary concern is with the function of the social worker as a member of the rehabilitation team. In this capacity her interest centers on the patient's personal and social adjustment as it affects his acceptance or rejection of rehabilitation plans. Since she is dealing with the employment potentials of individuals suffering from irreversible pathology, additional demands are made upon her knowledge and skill.

One of the most important contributions the social worker can make is in arriving at an early assessment of the patient in order to determine his ability to profit by rehabilitation services as well as his willingness to accept them. The importance of such early case finding is essential if we are to prevent the deterioration that so frequently accompanies prolonged idleness and insure a successful adjustment. Armed with the understanding provided by an early comprehensive study of the patient's cultural background, his role in the family and in the community, his social and emotional needs, his attitude toward his illness and disability, and the way in which his usual pattern of behavior and normal satisfactions is affected by it, and by the restrictions it imposes, the social worker can help with those social and personal problems which block the patient's acceptance of the rehabilitation program, and minimize whatever frustrations arise as a result of delays or changes in plans. Aware of the patient's attitudes toward what he considers to be interference with previously set goals, his fear of loss of personal worth, his lack of security, and his temporarily increased dependency, she can minimize destructive attitudes and support the undamaged part of the individual's personality. She can provide such alternate satisfactions as may be indicated and practicable, and set reasonable goals in the light of existing limitations.

Accepting the patient's level of functioning, giving him recognition for his achievements as he overcomes the difficulties as may arise at different stages of the process, expressing confidence in his ability for future development, the social worker can help to minimize what appear to be insurmountable aspects of the patient's handicap and in this way make each experience a positive step toward the attainment of the eventual goal.

The sick person in a hospital is often seen as being isolated from his social milieu. In reality, however, the patient is part of a wider world, a world of family, friends, and social group to which he returns upon leaving the hospital. Recognizing that the attitude of those close to the patient influences his own attitude toward his handicap and his readiness to accept and profit by the rehabilitation services offered him, the social worker has an important role to play in securing the family's participation, in preserving family unity, and in utilizing the strength inherent in familial bonds. Accomplishment of this result may necessitate the rendering of direct help to family members, by emphasizing the patient's strengths and securing their assistance in helping the patient in his efforts to reduce the extent of his handicap and achieve a satisfactory adjustment.

Because the patient's remaining disability may interfere with a resumption at his previous functioning level, environmental situations frequently have to be altered to remove such barriers as may exist. At other times the problems which arise require for their solution the combined help of organized community facilities. The social worker can help through an imaginative utilization of all available resources and by spearheading movements to fill the gaps.

The social worker has an obligation, as do the other team members, to share her understanding of the patient and his life situation and to integrate her thinking with that of the other professionals. These areas, dealing with study, treatment, and communication, comprise the social worker's primary contribution to the common goal.

The teamwork process, as here outlined, calls for more than an exchange of knowledge, or a summation of information gathered by the team members, or even a combination of skills. It means an integration of the knowledge and skills of the participating professions in such a way that it cross-fertilizes the contribution of each and gives added depth to their understanding of the patient and his problems.

SHELTERED WORKSHOPS

The present practice of shorter hospitalizations means that patients must sometimes leave the hospital before rehabilitation efforts have achieved their objective, and a continuation of these efforts following the patient's return to the community may be indicated. Experience has demonstrated that in such instances a period in a sheltered workshop can be utilized constructively, as a transition between hospital and community living and to maintain the gains secured through a well-planned and integrated program initiated in the hospital. Such an experience, it was found,

completes the medical service, prevents the loss of gains which have been made physically and mentally, and continues improvement physically, mentally, and socially towards a maximum of recovery and re-adjustment. It is the bridge between disability and illness and physical and mental health, between hospital environment and the obligations and associations of social and community life.[18]

What is a "sheltered workshop" or, as it is sometimes called, a "curative," "rehabilitative," "occupational," or "industrial" center? The Fair Labor Standards Act of 1938 defines a sheltered workshop as "a charitable organization or institution conducted not for profit, but for the purpose of carrying out a recognized program of rehabilitation for individuals whose earning capacity is impaired by age or physical or mental deficiency or injury, and to provide such individuals with remunerative employment or other occupational rehabilitating activity of an educational or therapeutic nature."

It is evident from this definition that the objectives of a sheltered workshop are not always the same, but depend upon the degree of the patient's recovery and the need for further restoration services. It can be used for some patients as a screening center, helping to determine realistically their employment potential through an evaluation of their work tolerance, abilities, interests, and capacities for meeting the physical and emotional demands of the job, as a basis for making an intelligent vocational choice. Those patients whose previous employment is no longer suitable, in view of their disability, or who had never acquired any particular skill, can train for a new occupation in a sheltered workshop. Because of the meaning of work and the importance which the ability to be self-maintaining assumes in our culture, the return of a handicapped person to productive employment is often thought to be the most important contribution made by a sheltered workshop.

Another group in the sheltered workshop is composed of patients whose disability makes it impossible for them at the time of discharge from the hospital to work more than a few hours a day, but who can look to an eventual return to nor-

[18] Elton, p. 4.

mal employment and can profit by a "hardening" or "conditioning" process which bring them to their maximum work tolerance, and slowly prepares them for outside employment.

Finally, there are those patients whose handicap precludes the possibility of returning to competitive industry and for whom a sheltered workshop is a place where they can remain indefinitely, sometimes permanently, learning a new and different way of living. Even though this represents the maximum working capacity they can achieve, the fact that they are profitably engaged often helps them to retain a feeling of usefulness and is conducive to a better social and emotional adjustment. However, if we are to safeguard the constructive utilization of the sheltered workshop on such an indefinite basis, it is important to insure that it is not used merely as a means for meeting the patient's dependency needs or for escape from reality when a different plan would serve his welfare better.

The objectives of the sheltered workshop, as expressed by one of its earliest exponents, are based on the experience of the Altro Workshops in New York City, organized in 1913 for the rehabilitation of the tuberculous and later expanded to provide similar services for cardiacs and the emotionally disturbed. These objectives, as stated by its former director, Edward Hochhauser—"Sheltered workshops for the physically handicapped, through productive, graduated work, with medical and social care and supervision, have as their objectives the physical, psychological and social adjustment of the patient" [19]—remain valid today.

To attain these objectives, it is important that the sheltered workshop meet certain fundamental prerequisites. First, in keeping with present-day thinking, the approach to the patient must be individualized; that is, it must rest on an evaluation of the patient's total personality, on his previous

[19] Hochhauser, p. 533.

work experience, and the extent to which the illness and resultant disability interfere with his work capacity both physically and emotionally.

The second prerequisite is the provision of a variety of services as an essential part of the program. Since we are here dealing with individuals handicapped by a residue of their illness, continued medical supervision and drug therapy as indicated are indispensable in order to maintain the gains achieved through medical care, enhance the patient's physical improvement, and provide such reassurance as he may need.

Not all patients react in the same way to a sheltered workshop experience. There are those for whom it may hold a real threat as a definite indication of their inability to resume an independent place in the community, or as perpetuation of a dependence which they resent and attempt to combat. The presence of a social worker thoroughly familiar with the program, working together with the other members of the staff, and sensitive to the patients' needs, can help them voice and overcome some of their feelings of helplessness and frustration and, by so doing, insure their cooperation.

For many of the patients who are to return to outside employment, the provision of vocational counseling and guidance is an essential part of the services of a sheltered workshop.

Thirdly, dealing with patients living in the community, the sheltered workshop cannot be an isolated function. It must be part of, and closely related to, the community to which they return.

The beneficial effects of a sheltered workshop experience have been demonstrated by a follow-up study of discharged patients conducted by the Altro Workshops. The report indicates that after a period of years, these patients show a reduction in relapses, improvement in physical and emotional well-being, and a resumption of economic usefulness through regaining old skills and acquiring new ones.[20]

[20] *Life and a Living.*

A later report of the follow-up of patients who were treated with antituberculosis drugs while undergoing a period of rehabilitation at Altro Workshops was published in 1956. The report shows that of 153 patients discharged during 1953–55, 104 were fully rehabilitated, 25 were partially rehabilitated, and 24 were not rehabilitated because of either recurring illness or psychological, social, or economic maladjustments.[21]

THE NEED FOR THE PATIENT'S ACTIVE PARTICIPATION

The patient is the center of rehabilitation activities, and any successful program must be based on his wholehearted participation in the efforts undertaken on his behalf:

Rehabilitation is not, and by its very nature cannot be, a matter of compulsion. There is no such thing as compelling a man to be rehabilitated. He can perhaps be compelled to go through certain motions and spend specified time at it, but it will be time and effort wasted unless there is the will to succeed.[22]

We must understand the factors which have a bearing on the patient's reaction to any step leading to greater self responsibility and remember that the individual functions as an integrated total personality. His disability is only one part of him. Besides the missing limb, the blind eye, the deaf ear, the injured lung, or the tired heart, there is a human being with a body otherwise undamaged and a mind which remains unaffected by the disease process. How he will react when faced with the prospect of greater self-responsiblity can be understood only in the light of his past experiences and his premorbid personality; for his past affects his present, and his present will influence his future. Illness, incapacity, and handicap can do no more than accentuate his normal behavior pattern; they do not change his intrinsic responses to situations. The aggressive and hostile patient will react in an aggressive way to any plan, no matter how appropriate it may be; the person who has achieved a reasonable degree of inde-

[21] Silzbach, p. 635.   [22] Sayer, p. 3.

pendence and maturity will respond to rehabilitation plans in an independent and mature way; the patient whose handicap and disability play into his need to be dependent, or who is fearful of facing life in the community because of his handicap, will not easily set forth on the road to greater independence.

A major difficulty which confronts every handicapped individual is the fact that he deviates from the normal. Cognizant of his inadequacies, incapable of competing on equal terms with the able-bodied, aware of the attitude of others toward him, the disabled person is likely to feel that he is "not as good" as other people, that he "does not measure up" to the standards of the group. In this, the patient's feelings about himself are reinforced by the attitude of people in the community; for there exists a widespread misconception that a handicap not only affects the particular area involved, but changes the whole person.

If the patient is to achieve a healthy adjustment, he must retain the conviction that the handicap does not devaluate him as a person; he must learn to recognize the limitations the disability imposes and set new goals in line with these limitations.

In our efforts to determine the level of functioning the patient can aspire to attain, it is important to keep in mind that the degree of disability involved is not in itself an indication of the extent of the handicap. The way the patient feels about his impairment, and about the frustrations it imposes, is of far greater importance. There are differentials in the impact of disability upon people. We all know patients who make astonishing progress despite what appear to be almost insurmountable physical difficulties, while others continue a vegetative existence even though the degree of physical impairment is minimal. There are those who prefer to wear out, and others who would rather rust out. Unless we learn to estimate the importance of the patient's emotional readiness to move from dependence to self-sufficiency, we may find that all the recent advances of scientific medicine and all the expanded community facilities will be of little avail in achieving the goal toward which our rehabilitation efforts are bent. The answer to the all-important question as to whether the patient will avail himself of the opportunity to learn more adequate functioning lies in the meaning illness has for him and the way in which we can help to strengthen positive attitudes and overcome negative ones. Our ability to motivate the patient toward undertaking tasks of increased complexity and to reduce feelings of frustration and helplessness will play an important role in the eventul success or failure of rehabilitation efforts.

IMPORTANCE OF REHABILITATION
AS PART OF MEDICAL CARE

At this point in our understanding of social welfare concepts, it is accepted that rehabilitation programs are an important part of total medical care for the chronically as well as the acutely ill.

These programs are based on the philosophy that in helping the patient to surmount his handicap, to overcome the deterioration which so often accompanies disuse, and to broaden his competence, no matter how minimal the achievement, we increase his feeling of worth and self-respect.

An effective rehabilitation program, which will enable us to accomplish this end, must include early planning, the provision of all medical facilities for diagnosis and treatment, the help of numerous professional disciplines in evaluating the patient's full potentials, and the inclusion of the patient in the total planning for his welfare. Whatever the ultimate objective may be, the immediate goal must at all times be set on a realistic level, that is, sufficiently high to have the patient feel that reaching it will represent an achievement and yet not so high as to expose him to possible failure and frustration. This implies that at no time can we think of rehabilitation goals as being static and definitively predetermined, but that they must be advanced gradually, as the patient meets one challenge after another. And finally, any program to be successful must be community-oriented and geared to meet the needs of the particular community within which it functions.

9

THE IMPACT OF ILLNESS ON THE FAMILY

ILLNESS AND SUFFERING have, since time immemorial, been matters of grave concern to all those who came into contact with them. The value attached to human life, the desire to prolong it and to alleviate suffering have through the centuries inspired the quest for ever more effective means of disease control and prevention.

We have come a long way from the early beginnings of the medicine man, not only in our technical skills but also in our understanding of patients as people. There is evidence of increasing recognition that in extending medical help and prolonging life we at the same time assume a responsibility to insure that the life which we succeed in prolonging is made more endurable, more fruitful, more satisfying.

Even this broadened goal of medical science, however, will fail to achieve its ultimate objective as long as we continue to confine our interest to the individual patient who comes to us for help. For the patient is not alone in his suffering; no patient is an isolated individual, no one lives in a vacuum. Through one relationship or another, he is tied to other individuals, and what disturbs him creates problems and difficulties for the many people comprising his circle. Like a pebble thrown into water, illness causes ever expanding circles, affecting not only the person who is ill but his family, which is called upon to meet many of the emotional and physical costs of the illness, his close relatives, and his friends.

In the course of the development of this broader interest and concern, our attention has shifted from the disease to the sick person, an integral part of a family group and a member of the society in which he lives.

EFFECT OF ILLNESS ON
FAMILY LIVING

Those most directly affected are members of the patient's immediate family, the group tied to him by bonds cemented through long years of living together. As Dr. H. B. Richardson so aptly expressed it, "the family is part of the individual and the individual is part of the family." [1] Having learned that "patients are people" and having accepted the axiom that "patients have families," we are now beginning to see the implications inherent in the fact that family members are people too. As people, they as well as the patient have feelings, ambitions, plans for the future. By virtue of the interaction existing between the members of the family group, these feelings, ambitions, and plans are not separate, distinct entities but are interrelated and interdependent. All of these may be, and often are, thwarted by the patient's illness.

What are the problems of greatest concern to the patient's family and how does it deal with them? Once again we find that no generalization can fit all cases. Families are but a composite of different individuals with different reactions. What these reactions will be, is determined by their own attitude to illness, the importance which the deprivations imposed have for them, and how long these deprivations have to be endured. Most important of all is the feeling they have about the patient, the place he holds in the family group, the outlook for the future, and how far it is possible to maintain the patient's status in the group. Furthermore, as is true with the patient, the problems which confront them vary with the

[1] Richardson, *Patients Have Families*, p. 68.

different stages of the illness, the degree to which it has progressed, and the amount of incapacity it produces.

The shock of the discovery of prolonged illness and its implications is as severe for family members as it is for the patient. The presence of a sick person in the home affects the life of the family, altering both its major aspects and the minutiae of everyday living.

If the patient is the man of the family and the bread-winner, the standards of living, plans for the future, and the entire tenor of life may have to be changed. Curtailment of income over a prolonged period of time, with no prospect of relief in sight, may impose hardships necessitating lowering of standards, readjustment in the pattern of living, and the need for other members of the family to assume the responsibilities once borne by the patient. Sometimes the wife may have to accept employment outside the home and either carry the burden of caring for the home while working, or make other plans for the supervision of the children. Even if the financial situation is such that the wife can continue in her traditional role of homemaker, if she is called upon to assume the additional task of caring for a sick man she may have little time, energy, or patience left for her home and children. We are all familiar with the undermining of physical resistance, increased tension, and irritability which this strain produces.

If the patient is the mother, all the effects of the temporary dislocation of family life seen in acute illness are intensified and multiplied. Even when the father or one of the children is able to act as a mother substitute, the usual pattern of living is often disrupted. The hastily prepared meals, frequently chosen because of the speed with which they can be put together rather than for their nutritive value, the inadequate care of the home, the very absence of the authority of the mother—all these affect the physical well-being of the family. What is more important is the change in the emotional tone of the home and the way in which all members of the family react to it.

The children feel the effects of prolonged illness in the home both directly and indirectly. Reduced income may mean abandonment of educational plans and consequent far-reaching implications for future life. In addition to the economic repercussions, more subtle effects are of equal significance. The whole life of the family may revolve around the sick person. The attention his condition requires and the concern about his welfare may deprive the children of the care to which they have been accustomed and which is essential for their development. Their interests, their problems and joys which were of paramount importance to their parents may of necessity be relegated to a secondary place. The fact that one of their parents is sick may determine what they eat and when, whether they go for a walk or attend a movie, whether they can secure a restful night of sleep. What will be the reaction of the school-age son who is late to class because his father's illness kept the household up all night? Or that of the teen-age daughter who has to give up the birthday party she had planned for many months because of the distressing effect the expense and confusion may have on the parent?

Such disappointments may be more than the youngsters are able to accept. Add to this the anxiety, helplessness, and frustration that accompany the witnessing of another's suffering in the face of one's inability to alleviate the pain, the fear of contagion or inherited disease, the threat of death frequently inherent in the diagnosis itself, and we have, in some measure, a picture of the emotional plight in which families may find themselves. Sacrifices may be made willingly and gladly in the beginning, but as the stress of such demands continues over a long period of time the original concern for the welfare of the patient may be obscured, and replaced by bitterness and resentment. Whereas in the beginning, the children, identifying themselves with the parent's suffering, resented the illness, later they may come to resent the patient himself as well as the sacrifices his illness entails.

The strain and stress that illness imposes are inevitably reflected in the way the patient is treated by members of his family group. Fearful of the illness and its implications, family members fight their natural desire to run away from day-to-day contact with it and the inexorable emotional strain it creates. Under pressure to do what they feel is expected of them, they are often overzealous in their efforts on the patient's behalf, suppressing what they really feel. When a person remains sick for a long time, his family in its concern about the illness tends to forget the person who is sick. They see him surrounded by an aura of "goodness" that may be completely different from what he actually is and what they know him to be. Very often, the patient becomes "the little man upon the stair who wasn't there." We are all familiar with the sickroom voice, the sickroom manner, and the inclination to protect the patient from any unpleasantness from the outside world. This creates an artificial atmosphere charged with the tension of unrelenting effort to suppress the unconsidered word, the irritable reaction. Such protection often springs from a natural feeling that the patient is "too sick to be bothered." Well-meaning as such overprotectiveness may be, to the patient it means exclusion; for it cuts him off from the good and bad, joys and sorrows, that constitute everyday living. It serves as a denial of his rights as a family member. The fact that he is a passive onlooker on the day-to-day life of the family group acts as a constant reminder of his own uselessness, displacement, and inadequacy. In an effort to assert his importance, the patient may revert to a type of behavior which, unless understood, may be difficult to cope with. He may complain, or demand demonstrations of attention and affection, creating a situation fraught with danger both for himself and for all those around him.

In other instances, the overprotectiveness may be but a way of controlling the sick person, the inclination to control being evoked by the patient's very helplessness. The net result is that the patient is robbed of his right to have a say in how his life, whatever remains of it, is to be lived. Such an exclusion and the feeling of rejection it can engender may well undermine the patient's will to live and, consequently, his response to medical treatment. We have seen, in the case of Mr. W., how his inclusion in family living, his participation in family problems, was utilized as a help not only in combating his illness, but in reestablishing his feeling of worth as an individual.

If the work with Mr. W. and others like him is not to go for naught, families too need to be helped to understand what the patient's individual needs are and how their ability to meet these needs may influence the actual course of his illness. In doing this we must keep in mind that members of the family are individuals too, with needs, desires, strivings, and that the patient's illness may, and often does, interfere with the satisfactions they seek. Merely suppressing these needs or denying their existence is no solution of their problem. If anything, such constant suppression builds up a reservoir of frustration which is bound to explode sooner or later, to the detriment of all concerned.

As we try to envisage all it may mean to those concerned, we began to realize that it is no small burden family members are called upon to carry. There are limits to human endurance.

REACTION OF THE FAMILY
TO HOSPITALIZATION

A time may come when the demands of the patient's condition make continued care in the home impractical and his

removal to the hospital the only means of securing the necessary medical care.

The meaning of hospitalization to family members can be
best understood if we keep in mind the community's attitude
towards hospitalization in general and admission to a hospital
for "chronic disease" in particular. In the past, patients
entered such hospitals to die. Community attitudes change
slowly, and relatives still react with fear, anxiety, and often
guilt to the implication that in arranging for hospitalization
they are in reality "putting the sick person away." There are
instances where this feeling is so intense that relatives resist
taking such a step, thus depriving the patient of whatever
benefits he might derive from hospital care. At other times,
the decision may be arrived at only after a long and painful
struggle, and only when circumstances leave no alternative.
Even after a decision has been reached the implications
inherent in the need for hospitalization, the seriousness of
the patient's condition, and the worry about the eventual
outcome create problems which are real and severe.

Despite the difficulties in caring for a sick person in the
home, his removal does not eliminate probems for his
family; it merely shifts the focus of their concern. While the
patient was in the home the family may have had the heavy
physical burden of caring for him, and the emotional burden
of watching his suffering. Now, his very absence, the anxiety
about his condition from hour to hour, may create an
atmosphere of tension with resulting disorganization and
purposeless, frenzied activity, as if by such activity the family
can fill the gap. The whole routine of family living may
become centered on hospital visiting hours, requiring adjustments in their accustomed routine which may not come
easily.

Because of the atmosphere of illness, suffering, and death
traditionally associated with hospitals, family members as
well as patients react with fear and misgivings. They too are

awed by the unfamiliar surroundings and bewildered by the impersonal routine. While the patient, uncomfortable and fearful though he may be, knows at least how he is feeling and, in part, what is happening to him, family members are left in the dark and can only feed on their own fears and anxieties, continuing at the same time to cope with the many hardships his illness creates in the home. Beset by these numerous problems, they may feel left out in the cold as they see all the care and attention lavished on the patient.

We have discussed previously the fear of incapacity, suffering, and death which haunts the patient. Family members, tied as they are to the patient emotionally, react to the same fears. Let us take the diagnosis of cancer, for example. Even though an attempt is made by the doctor to keep the knowledge of the diagnosis from the patient, family members are usually told the nature of the illness. This means that when subjected to questioning by the patient, they are forced to be secretive and evasive, fearful lest in an unguarded moment they may let the patient learn what they know. Under the stress of their own anxiety, they react with tension and need help not only to relieve such tension, but also to learn how to handle the patient's questions.

It frequently happens that both the patient and members of the family are aware of the nature of the illness, but do not dare to speak of it openly because each tries to shield the other. When they are together during visiting hours they try to be cheerful and keep away from discussing what is really troubling them so as to spare each other's feelings. How much this restraint costs them is evidenced by the fact that often both the patient and the relatives seek out the social worker following visiting hours in order to discuss their doubts, misgivings, and fears, as the only means of release from the tension under which they labor.

Because of the dread associated with cancer, family members may need help with problems which the illness poses for them. Cancer, like many other illnesses whose origin is still unknown, often raises questions in their minds about heredity, familial predisposition, and contagion. They need to be encouraged, not only to bring these questions into the open but also to enable them to get realistic reassurance by submitting to a medical examination.

The fear of contagion, when it is realistic, as it is when tuberculosis is involved creates other problems with far-reaching implications. The medical surveillance of family members, necessary as it is to check the spread of the disease, not surpising that the well spouse sometimes becomes bitter and bitterness. These feelings, combined with prolonged separation and economic insecurity, frequently threaten the very continuation of the pattern of family living.

In other instances, the primary problem centers on the hopelessness of the medical condition and the probability of permanent invalidism. It is true that in any serious illness the spouse may be confronted with the possibility of a fatal prognosis. When this happens, and traumatic as such an experience may be, some adjustment is eventually achieved and a new patten of life established. Not so in the progressive degenerative conditions. Here the marital partner may have to face the prospect of being saddled with a hopeless invalid for an indefinite period of time. This may mean assumption of the double role of father and mother, being the provider while at the same time carrying the responsibility for the home and children without any relief in sight. It is not only accentuates the fear but may give rise to resentment and vents his anger on the patient, whose very helplessness seemingly provokes and encourages expressions of hostility.

In some instances the hostility is undisguised. Nobility of character has its limits. The marital partner may utilize the visiting hours either to complain about hardships or to emphasize the ability to manage alone. In either event, the patient, feeling helpless to cope with the situation or to affect it in any way, reacts with superficial acceptance of the fact that "he does not matter any more." In other instances, the hostility is expressed indirectly through infrequent visits, unwillingness to have the patient come home on a pass, or refusal to bring the children to visit him. The net result in either case is that the patient feels rejected, "left out," excluded from normal participation in family living. It can be readily seen that such treatment of the patient and his reaction to it would seriously affect the manner in which he would respond to medical treatment. The importance of the patient's willingness to continue the fight for life has long been recognized by the medical profession.

FAMILY MEMBERS NEED HELP

Recognizing that the attitude of family members is an important element, facilitating or retarding the patient's progress, it devolves upon those concerned with his care to help them handle some of these problems so that they may find release and not be forced to vent their feelings upon the patient. Experience has shown that the same methods which have proved effective in helping the patient can be applied as successfully in dealing with members of his family. As with the patient, working with family members implies a willingness to recognize and help with the problems rather than a denial that such problems exist. They need sustained help, recognition of the burden they are called upon to carry, and an opportunity to voice their frustration and grievances. The best results are obtained with inclusion, not exclusion, of family members in planning for the patient's care. With an opportunity to participate actively in the therapeutic measures instituted by the medical team on the patient's behalf, they can become understanding, sympathetic, and useful adjuncts in treatment. Unfortunately, however, the busy routine of a hospital provides but small opportunity for such active working together. Relatives feel, and rightly so, that the patient's physician is their most reliable source of information. In reality, however, relatives seldom succeed in seeing the doctor and often find it difficult to understand the implications of the patient's illness or to obtain reliable information about his physical condition. Theoretically, doctors are available to members of the family during visiting hours; actually, they are seldom in evidence, being busy elsewhere. If and when the relatives succeed in finding a doctor to answer their questions, privacy and sufficient time are often lacking so that many of the questions that trouble them remain unasked and unanswered. In most instances, they perforce have to be satisfied with the stock replies from the information desk that "the patient is as well as can be expected," or "is resting comfortably." These may sound reassuring, but they certainly fail to answer the numerous questions relatives have in mind, and leave them with a sense of helplessness and frustration.

When these unanswered questions persist, as they usually do, the mounting anxiety and tension are inevitably reflected in the emotional tone of the visits. Presumably, visiting hours are a means of maintaining the patient's contact with those close to him and thus bolster his morale. A relative who is anxious, fearful, and tense, who sits at the bedside with one eye constantly on the corridor trying to catch sight of a doctor, communicates his restlessness to the patient and by so doing negates the beneficial effect of his visit.

FAMILY NIGHT

The mounting difficulties created by this situation, the dissatisfaction expressed by doctors, patients, and relatives alike, led to the institution of "Family Night" at Montefiore Hospital in New York in 1948.[2] A special hour, immediately preceding the visiting hours, was set aside each week to give

[2] Field, "Family Sessions—a New Cooperative Step in a Medical Setting," pp. 417-21.

families an opportunity to discuss matters freely with the professional team concerned with the patient's care—the doctor and the social worker. These sessions, variously referred to as "Family Night," "Interviewing Night," or "Tuesday Night Clinic," steadily gained in popularity. Ever larger numbers of members of patients' families availed themselves of the opportunity for free and unhurried discussion of the problems which illness posed for them.

As was to be expected, the questions raised for discussion were many and varied. They differed widely, depending upon the nature of the illness the social, economic, and emotional problems the illness created for the patient and the family, and the relationships within the family group. The question most frequently heard was: "What is the matter with the patient?" All too often the doctor, taking the question at its face value, gave the diagnosis. While it is true that the relatives wanted to know the name of the illness, the diagnosis did not seem to provide the information they were really seeking, or answer the questions they had in mind. In most instances, the name itself, even when translated into lay terminology, means little, for the average layman does not have enough medical knowledge to appraise its significance or connotation. Under pressure of their own anxieties, family members may react to the implication of hopelessness it conveys to them, fear the worst, and ignore the real potentialities for meaningful living the patient retains. When a member of the family asks, "What is the matter with the patient?" he is really asking not only for the name of the illness but for a prognosis as well. He wants to know what the future holds, what he can expect. It is only as the medical diagnosis is supplemented by an interpretation of its social implications that it takes on meaning for those concerned with the patient's welfare. It is then that the patient emerges, not merely as a disease entity, but as a functioning human being with strengths as well as weaknesses, potentialities as well as limitations. The frightening aspects of the patient's illness lose some of their terror as the relatives realize that the illness itself is but one part of the total picture, that it does not change the patient, that he remains a human being— with limitations, it is true, but retaining many of the strengths he had before he became ill.

Despite the physical removal from the home, despite the separation of hospital existence from everyday community living, the patient maintains ties with his family group and his social circle. Interaction between patient and family continues even though physical contact is limited to visiting hours. As the patient is subjected to different treatment procedures, new drugs, or special diets, as these raise questions in his mind, he is likely to convey his concern to members of his family. They, in turn, may find it difficult to evaluate objectively the patient's complaints about diet, nursing care, medical attention, restrictions, the general hospital routine. They may find it difficult to understand that such complaints are but a reflection of the patient's total reaction to being ill, uncomfortable, and unhappy, or to appreciate his need to attribute his unhappiness to externals. In their concern for the patient's welfare it is easy for them to accept his complaints at face value and, by so doing, fortify his belief that he is being neglected or ill-treated. Given an opportunity to raise these questions with the doctor and to understand the underlying reasons for the medical restrictions and recommendations, relatives were able not only to withstand the pressures exerted by the patient, but to become active and useful allies of the professional team caring for him.

There comes to mind a mild little woman who came to see the doctor during Family Night. Her question was extremely simple. Her husband complained that he did not get oranges, she said. She could understand that perhaps the hospital could not afford to supply them. Would it be all right for her to bring some every time she came to visit?

The doctor explained that this was not a matter of economy. Oranges were not given to this particular patient because he was on a special diet. Perhaps she could help by explaining it to the patient. The woman's face lit up. "Of course I will," she said. "He will take it from me. He knows I would not deny him oranges."

In this simple way, a short discussion with the doctor helped to make a valuable ally of the patient's wife in rendering the necessary medical care.

As the relatives discussed the patient's situation with the doctor and social worker many aspects of the family relationships, hitherto unknown, came to light. This helped the doctor to understand the emotional atmosphere in which the patient lived prior to his illness and to which he would eventually return. Changes that needed to be made could then be undertaken, not as something imposed upon the patient and the family from without, but as part of a plan arrived at jointly in which the relatives participated actively and the purpose of which they understood. Such active participation helps the family accept the restrictions imposed by the illness and the readjustments it may require with greater ease. Family Night interviews have proved to be of value not only to the patients and their families, but also to the professional people concerned with the patients' care.

These joint sessions provided an opportunity to observe the interplay between the patient and his family and the effect of the emotional and familial components on the patient's physical condition. The patient ceased to be merely a "sick person"; instead, he was seen as a total human being. The family was no longer something separate from the patient, but became an integral and essential part of the team whose primary function was to preserve the values achieved through extensive hospital care.

The Family Night program was originally instituted for the benefit of those patients whose families did not have a private physician to whom they could address their questions. In 1961 a new building was added to the hospital. Special wards were abolished, making it possible to end the segregation of ward patients and to have them share the facilities with the semiprivate group. The house staff was thus able to see family members during regular visiting hours, and the Family Night program was therefore discontinued in May of that year.

REACTION OF THE FAMILY
TO THE PATIENT'S RETURN HOME

Difficult as the period of hospitalization may be, all problems for the family do not end when the patient returns home. Because of the nature of prolonged illness, in many instances a discharge recommendation may mean that the family has to take home a patient whose condition shows but little change, and who requires a type of care which the family feels unable to provide. They often react to such a recommendation with confusion and bewilderment.

Such confusion is understandable if we bear in mind what we have said earlier about the problems families face at point of admission. For those who saw in hospitalization the "last stepping stone" and who have, after a severe inner struggle, decided to "put the patient away," the prospect of his return home may be as much of a shock as was the necessity of his being hospitalized. Having gone through the struggle, having worked through their guilt, they are suddenly faced with the realization that the situation has altered but slightly, if at all, and that they are called upon to assume responsibility once again.

On the other hand, those who viewed hospitalization with hope may find that the improvement is but slight and that difficult as the hospitalization period was for them, it failed to accomplish what they had expected of it. Under such circumstances it is natural that their concern is primarily not with new concepts of medical treatment or new trends in hospital care, but rather with what the patient's return home will mean to him and to them personally. What troubles them most is the question of what they are to do about the problems which the residue of the illness may cause. In this, their concern is realistic, for the sequelae of prolonged illness often extend beyond the hospitalization and may continue to exert their influence not only on the patient's physical condition, but on his entire pattern of living, affecting his economic security, his relationship with his family, and his feelings about himself for a long time to come, or even indefinitely. Under these circumstances, it is not surprising to find that difficulties are frequently encountered when it is necessary to discharge a patient who is obviously incapable of resuming his normal role in the family and the community.

When the patient is a child who is handicapped by the residue of his illness, the family may have equally difficult problems. The condition of the patient, requiring extra care, may make him the center of family life, monopolize the parents' time to the exclusion of the needs of siblings, and thus alter the entire pattern of family living.

Such concentrated care, even though considered essential for the welfare of the patient, may affect the behavior of the other children. Feeling deprived, they may react with types of behavior which express their dissatisfaction and serve to regain some of the parents' attention. It is indeed not easy to strike a balance between the time to be devoted to the sick child and to the needs of the other children, or to devise means for including the sick child in the life of the family.

MAKING A HOME FOR THE PATIENT

Sometimes realistic difficulties, such as crowded conditions, complete absence of a home, or the illness or frailty of the spouse, stand in the way of releasing the patient from the hospital. At other times, the real difficulty in effecting discharge lies in the underlying rejection of the patient by his family, such obstacles as are set up being merely devices to cloak the rejection.

Particular problems arise in arranging for the discharge of the older patient who, having no home of his own, must of necessity depend on his children. In a society built on the strength of the family as a unit, the obligation of children to care for their parents is sometimes taken for granted. Into it go the accepted concepts of gratitude, filial devotion, repayment of debt, and the like. And yet if we are to maintain and protect the family unit, we must consider what the carrying out of this obligation may do to the preservation of the new family units the grown children themselves establish. Sometimes it happens that because of the tendency to associate prolonged illness with the need for permanent institutionalization, the hospitalization of an elderly parent is interpreted as a custodial placement. This may precipitate the breaking up of the home, with the other parent going to live with the children. When the patient is ready to return home, he finds that the home is no longer there. The married children, having made arrangements for one parent, may find it difficult to include the other at the time when the hospital is ready to discharge him. Even when the children are willing to take the patient, necessary stair climbing in their home, scarcity of space, or the objections of the marriage partners may present valid practical difficulties.

Or the children may be unwilling to accept an old and ailing parent into their home, fearing the added burden, the physical and emotional responsibility they are asked to assume, and the effect his presence will have on their own family life. The curtailment of privacy, the necessary readjustments in family living, the additional burden of physical care and the emotional burden of witnessing suffering, unpleasant sights and odors, and the ever present specter of impending death, not as a groundless fear but as a part of reality—all are important factors which need to be taken into consideration. Whether children can be asked to assume such a burden must be evaluated in the light of existing family ties and the danger of disrupting family living. All these factors are important. They form the warp and woof of living and cannot be dismissed lightly. They must be weighed carefully with due recognition that there is no easy solution to the problems they pose.

Important and real as are these various factors in some instances, in others they merely serve to cloak the family's unwillingness to make a home for the patient. Underlying this unwillingness one finds discord, irritation, and rejection accumulated during years of living together. It is to be expected that these feelings, more or less successfully covered up, should forcibly come to the surface at the time of discharge. The neglect of the patient in the hospital, failure to visit him or to evince interest, can be ascribed to lack of time, distance from the home, preoccupation with other duties. These rationalizations can no longer be used when the family is faced with the prospect of an imminent return home.

PROBLEMS CREATED BY THE PATIENT'S PRESENCE

Even when family members are eager to have the patient at home, they may find that the limitations imposed by the illness demand a rearrangement in their pattern of living which is difficult to achieve. The problem is further aggravated by the fact that such changes in family living have to be made with the knowledge that it is not a temporary expedient but may have to be continued indefinitely. Harassed by the problems the patient's presence creates, they may find that they have little understanding of his needs and less patience in coping with them. They frequently need interpretation of the limitations created by the residual aspects of the illness and the importance of continuing some of the routines to which the patient was subjected while in the hospital. The very freedom of the home makes it difficult for the patient to follow the rules laid down by the physician. It becomes even more difficult for him if the relatives, in their eagerness to lead as normal a life as possible, urge the patient to forget his diet or to stay up late "just this once" for a special occasion.

Recognizing how difficult may be the readjustments required, it is not surprising to find that having made whatever arrangements were necessary and possible for the patient's comfort, having sacrificed a great deal of their personal freedom to provide for his needs, relatives may be unable to understand why the patient should be dissatisfied or unhappy. They question what else they can or should do to alleviate this unhappiness and they find no satisfactory answer. After a while, their natural concern for the patient's welfare becomes tinged with impatience and irritability. The situation becomes further complicated because of the emotional problems of the family members themselves; for the very process of making allowances for the patient often means a suppression of their own emotional needs. It is essential for the welfare both of the patient and of his family that help be given them in facing their problems.

Where the family ties are strong and there is evidence of a genuine concern for the welfare of the patient, members of the family respond readily when the contribution they are making to promote the patient's well-being is given adequate recognition. The services they are rendering can become in themselves a source of satisfaction. Where the family ties of affection and concern are weak, there often occurs a rivalry situation because of the attention the sick member gets and irritation because of his uselessness and dependence. With our concern centered primarily on the sick person, we are in danger of forgetting that members of the family too are individuals, the satisfaction of whose emotional needs is constantly being interfered with by the presence of a sick and handicapped person. While it may be difficult or even impossible to provide alternate satisfactions, a thorough understanding of, and sympathy with, the problem and concrete assistance in carrying the burden has proved to be helpful in the past. Greater consciousness of the severity of the problem, which until now has not received adequate recognition, will aid us to develop better skills in its handling.

Even the discharge of patients to a program of home care, with all the services that this implies, does not prevent difficulties from arising. Since the rendering of medical care in the home is dependent for its success on the active cooperation of members of the patient's family, ways and means have to be devised to give them the necessary assisttance in carrying out their responsibilities. Such help can be given only if we have a thorough appreciation of the problems which the reality of the situation poses for the family, and the difficulties, both physical and emotional, to which it may give rise. No matter how strong the family ties, or how genuine the desire to help the patient, the prospect of having a seriously sick person in the home is bound to arouse tensions, fears, and anxieties. The problems created by the discharge of patients suffering from prolonged illness have been pointed out earlier. Here we have the additional problems inherent in the fact that we are sending home a patient who is admittedly in need of continued intensive medical supervision. Families whose relative is in the hospital may react to the uncertainty about his physical condition from hour to hour. The presence of a sick person in the home is likely to foster a different kind of anxiety and frustration arising from the recognition of their helplessness in the face of discomfort, pain, and suffering. Under these circumstances, it is natural that families should question their ability to stand the strain, even with the help the program can provide.

To insure against unreasonable expectations and subsequent disappointments, family members need to understand clearly the service the program can provide as well as what their contribution is to be, how much care the patient will require, and how much he can be expected to do for himself. Even when given the most careful interpretation, however, many families find it difficult to believe that the interest of the hospital will be maintained following the patient's physical removal from the institution. They require a period of testing, to convince themselves that their problems will be met, before they can feel secure and relaxed. It is only as they see the application of the program to their particular situation that it takes on meaning for them. The simple services the hospital stands ready to render—providing a hospital bed or hospital equipment as needed; sending in a dentist if the patient has a toothache; arranging for a nurse to visit soon after the patient gets home—mean more to the family than all the explanations of the program we can give them, for they represent solid evidence of the hospital's continued interest.

There was, for instance, John, a boy of 19. The mother, aware that the boy had cancer in an advanced stage, and realizing that little could be done for him medically, was eager to have him home. He would be more comfortable and happier at home than in the hospital, she said. She could wait on him, show him love and attention.

She was, however, worried a little, she admitted. She was told that the doctor would visit, but what was she to do in an emergency? And suppose he got one of those "spells" which made breathing so difficult? What was she to do? When it was explained that a hospital bed and oxygen could be provided in the home, that she could call for a doctor whenever she felt it necessary, she relaxed somewhat. It was apparent, however, that all her questions had not been answered and that there remained an underlying fear that she would be left alone to face an emergency.

The first few weeks following John's discharge, his mother telephoned almost daily. Requests for the doctor to call were frequent, as were her requests for advice from the social worker even on minor problems. It was only when she became convinced through actual experience that her calls would be answered that she was able to adhere to a definite schedule of visits. At the same time, the frequency of her calls to the social worker diminished. Slowly she regained her capacity to deal with problems unaided.

Even though little could be done to shield her from the shock of losing her son, she was able to derive some satisfaction from the knowledge that she "had done her duty" by her son by caring for him to the very end.

Because of the magnitude of the responsibility which devolves upon them, family members need support, reassurance, and help throughout the patient's illness in the home. Above all else, they need evidence of understanding, appreciation, and approval for the difficult job they are doing and an opportunity to voice their doubts, questionings, and, at times, discouragement without being made to feel that by complaining they are derelict in their duty.

INCLUDING THE PATIENT IN FAMILY LIVING

One of the greatest difficulties which family members encounter lies in the necessity to alter established behavior patterns to include the incapacitated patient and to help him preserve the new values he has built up for himself. Such an adjustment is often not easy to make. If we agree that patterns of behavior are developed to satisfy emotional needs, then change can take place only if the satisfactions the behavior provided are replaced by other satisfactions. Where the family group is a cohesive unit and where the patient is genuinely accepted and loved, the concern for his welfare can be utilized as a base on which to build a new pattern of family living and sharing. When the family ties are not strong, when there is a backlog of accumulated resentment, such substitution is difficult and sometimes impossible.

Even under the most favorable circumstances, family members as well as the patient may have to go through a difficult period of adjustment in learning to live together with a minimum of friction and some degree of satisfaction. We have learned through years of experience that family members respond in a very positive way to their being included in direct and active participation in the care of the patient. In the course of such planning, the patient begins to emerge as a distinct individual. Once the family begins to see that illness and disability do not detract from the patient's worth, they may be helped to avail themselves of the contribution he can make to family living, a contribution which is a source of strength for them and satisfaction to him. How this has been accomplished in one instance, is illustrated by the story of Mrs. H.:

During the time Mrs. H. was in the hospital, Mr. H. took over the mother role and gave the children excellent supervision. As the time for the patient's discharge from the hospital approached, Mr. H. made plans to have a part-time maid, since he knew that Mrs. H. would be confined to a wheel chair at least for a while after her return home.

When Mrs. H. was seen shortly after her discharge and was asked whether she was able to get sufficient rest now that she was home, her reply was: "Sure I rest. What is there for me to do? The maid does the heavy work. My husband waits on me hand and foot. He has taken complete charge. He plans, he supervises the children. He is a good husband." Behind these words of praise and appreciation one could detect an all-pervading sense of hopelessness and uselessness.

Mr. H., when the situation was discussed with him, mentioned his wife's lack of interest in what was going on around her. She was so apathetic, he said, nothing interested her. She seemed to have withdrawn into a shell.

His concern about her lack of interest was recognized as valid and he was drawn into planning ways and means to get Mrs. H. to participate in the life of the family, make her feel a part of what was going on around her, and even assume some responsibility. Mrs. H.'s physical condition was discussed in detail to clarify for her huband what she was able to do as well as what was beyond her physical strength at that point.

Little by little, Mr. H. was given help in understanding that despite the patient's inability to perform physical tasks, she could still maintain her place in the household by continuing to direct and supervise the conduct of the home and the children. As his conviction grew that this responsibility would actually help in his wife's recovery, Mr. H. was able to relinquish some of the controls he had taken over. Under his guidance the children learned once more to turn to their mother for their weekly allowances, to have their hair combed before going to school, and to bring their homework and report cards to her when they returned home.

Realizing how much the loss of this close tie with the children meant to Mr. H., and how much he was asked to relinquish for the sake of the patient's welfare, the social worker tried to devise means to compensate him for this deprivation. She involved him in an appraisal of how Mrs. H. was responding to this new regime, and gave him recognition for the personal sacrifices he was making in his efforts to help her. Rewarded by this appreciation of his contribution to the change in Mrs. H.'s reactions, and her increased interest in what was going on around her, Mr. H. was able to take the next step and to consult her about planning meals and the general running of the home.

Thus the satisfaction he derived from being in complete charge of his home was replaced by the satisfaction of being the one who was responsible for the improvement Mrs. H. was showing. He learned that in spite of her handicap, Mrs. H. remained an individual who had a contribution to make to the life of the family and who could derive normal satisfactions in feeling that she had a share in the family's well-being.

In other instances, the very plan for the patient to remain in the home hinges upon the care taken to prevent family disruption through placing too heavy a burden upon the other members. While it is essential for the patient to receive the attention he requires, it does not necessarily mean that every member of the family must constantly and completely sacrifice all his personal needs and desires. Indeed, there are times when such sacrifices merely serve to accentuate the patient's feeling of being a burden:

In the case of Mrs. N., previously cited, the patient felt her uselessness so keenly that she preferred to go to a custodial institution rather than be a burden to her children.

The welfare of this patient and her ability to remain under the home care program did not depend exclusively on the help she was to receive from her children. On the contrary, it was essential that the children be given an understanding of the patient's need to be not only independent but helpful to others. In the light of such an understanding the children's willingness to forego all their personal needs and devote themselves completely to the patient in reality negated all the good they tried to accomplish.

In order to help both them and the patient, the children were encouraged to allow her to do as much as she could possibly manage, regardless of their desire to help her at all times. They were urged to turn to her for help in small matters, increasing her responsibilities, step by step, as her condition allowed.

Since Mrs. N. complained that her presence kept her children tied to the house and robbed them of recreation, the children were helped to arrange a schedule which would assure that Mrs. N. was not left alone, while at the same time allowing the other members of the family to lead as normal a life as possible.

The two cases cited represent an excellent adjustment on the part of all concerned. It would be unrealistic to expect that such results can always be achieved. However, even when the situation is such that actually we can accomplish little, we can, as long as we maintain a regard for the realistic difficulties inherent in the situation, relieve tension on the part of family members and to that extent make the patient's adjustment easier. Even when a satisfactory adjustment of the patient is impossible and his presence demands a difficult readjustment in the life of others, the family members often derive a certain amount of satisfaction from a duty fulfilled. As many of them phrase it, "At least there is nothing I can reproach myself for. I feel I have done all I could."

There is another area in which help is sometimes necessary. Our society imposes a moral obligation on families to care for their sick. If family members find themselves unable to carry out what they consider to be their obligation, they may react with feelings of guilt, tension, and resentment. Whatever their feeling, they are often unable to admit that they consider the care of the patient a burden, or that they wish to be relieved of it. The opportunity to discuss the problem with someone who is sympathetic, who does not hold them to a "performance of duty," who acknowledges that the situation is difficult and discouragement understandable, and who shares in plans for ways in which the burden can be lessened, provides a release from this sense of unbearable burden. Given such help, they can arrive at a decision as to whether they can continue caring for the patient, or whether other plans will need to be made. Whatever the final decision, they can make it on the basis of calm deliberation, a realistic appraisal of what is involved, rather than being prompted by emotions which they cannot express and of which they are but dimly aware.

10

A LONG-RANGE VIEW

OUR REVIEW of the problems that confront patients who suffer from prolonged illness shows all too clearly how extensively and intensively they affect every aspect of living both for the patient himself and for those closely associated with him. No situation is simple. Any attempt at a solution must take into consideration the numerous problems created by the interaction of individual attitudes and social, economic, and emotional factors. It is equally evident that in the past little could have been done to alleviate these problems because of scarcity of resources and the failure of the community to respond adequately to their urgency. As a result, no matter what aspect of prolonged illness we consider, we find that facilities for care are either completely lacking or are grossly inadequate to meet the needs.

RECOGNITION OF THE SERIOUSNESS
OF THE PROBLEM

If we agree that the primary objective for action in the field of public health is to prevent large-scale suffering and death, then prolonged illness with its toll of human suffering, its devastating effects on every aspect of personal, social, and even political living (if one considers the mental as well as the physical consequences), looms as public health problem Number One. Indeed, it represents a serious, if not the most serious, medical-social problem of our time.

The awareness of the importance of this problem becomes evident during the first half of the present century. Numerous articles in the professional and popular press are devoted to this subject with greater frequency; references to it are made in public speeches; it is discussed more and more frequently by organized hospital, medical, and nursing groups at professional gatherings. In 1947 a voluminous document, *Planning for the Chronically Ill*, was published through the combined efforts of the American Public Health Association, the American Medical Association, the American Hospital Association, and the American Public Welfare Association. The National Health Assembly devoted a whole section of its 1949 deliberations to a discussion of the implications of prolonged illness. The United States Congress passed several acts dealing with some of these specific prolonged illnesses, establishing the National Cancer Institute and the National Heart Institute. Federal funds were in some instances allocated to state public health departments for dealing with problems created by prolonged illness. Organizations to educate the public, to encourage research, and to combat the effects of specific prolonged illnesses were being organized on local and national levels. Newspapers, magazines, and radio commentators became increasingly vocal in their attempts to alert the public to the wide extent of prolonged illness, its implications, and the need for public support of treatment and research centers.

The widespread public interest and concern were hopeful signs. The history of medical progress reveals that the strides made in the fight against infectious and contagious diseases, such as smallpox, cholera, diphtheria, and malaria, came primarily as a response to the community's interest in these diseases spurred by the community's desire to protect itself against them. In this respect prolonged illness is at a disadvantage. Unlike the contagious diseases, prolonged illness, with few exceptions, like tuberculosis, cannot be communicated by personal contact, spread of germs, or inadequate sanitation. The devastation remains confined to the individual patient and for a long time was thought to affect directly only the patient himself and those who comprise his immediate circle.

It is only as the number of patients with prolonged illness increases that more and more people in the community are affected and gain at firsthand an understanding of the full impact of its ravages. This appreciation that as the span of life increases, our family, neighbors, and friends may all become likely targets for one of the crippling, disabling conditions known as prolonged illness should serve as an incentive to mobilize our resources, lift the problem from the narrow confines of the individual's concern, and see it as the public health menace it actually is.

In the absence of specific drugs to prevent the development of chronicity, hope lies in instilling an appreciation of the value of good health practices, periodic physical examinations, a greater awareness of the significance of early symptoms both by the medical profession and the public in general, general improvement of social and economic conditions of a large part of the population, and the availability and accessibility of high-quality medical care. It is only thus that we can anticipate strides in the conquest of the large host of prolonged illnesses now plaguing mankind commensurate with the advances made in the conquest of infectious and contagious diseases, the plagues of earlier centuries.

At present, however, we are still a long way from the attainment of such an objective. The statement made in 1933 that "the care of the chronic sick, in all of its phases, has been and is still a stepchild in the scheme of hospital organization" [1] still holds true.

In 1963 the Hospital Review and Planning Council of Southern New York found that "the critical shortage of ade-

[1] Hinenburg, p. 73.

quate and well-coordinated facilities and services for long term care is one of the most pressing problems of present time." [2]

While these statements emphasize the lack of hospital facilities, the inadequacies are duplicated in all other facilities which form part of a program of total medical care.

While we must admit that advances in the provisions for the care of patients with prolonged illness have been slow, nevertheless a beginning has been made. We no longer consign these patients to medical oblivion. The need for treatment is better understood, the inadequacy of treatment facilities is more widely recognized, and efforts to provide them are being made. Public attention is being focused on the necessity for improving, coordinating, and extending available facilities in every area concerned with prolonged illness. We are recognizing that the problems created by such illness extend beyond the medical needs, and that there is a close relationship between the patient's somatic disturbances, his social situation, and his emotional state. As a result our concern has shifted from the inadequate provision of purely custodial care or homes for the aged—on the assumption that prolonged illness is confined to the aged—to a type of care which encompasses the patient as an individual, an integral part of the family and the community. There is recognition of the need for prevention and research into causes—medical, social, and emotional—but, as is usually the case, facilities lag far behind our appreciation of the need.

METHODS OF
ATTACKING THE PROBLEM

Because of the multiplicity of areas of human living upon which prolonged illness impinges, any discussion of what can

[2] Hospital Review and Planning Council of Southern New York, Annual Report, 1963–1964, p. 20.

be done to attack the problem will necessarily involve many aspects. In some instances where the problems are similar to those created by acute illness, even though aggravated by the length of time over which they extend, we might profitably employ the same methods which have proved their efficacy in the past. It is important to remember, however, that there are additional problems created by the very prolonged nature of the illness and that these additional problems will, of necessity, demand new methods of attack.

A statement made by the Surgeon General of the United States Public Health Service gives concisely what should be done, if we are to help solve the numerous problems which prolonged illness creates for its victims and for the community. According to this statement, "a comprehensive plan for the care of the chronically ill must be based upon . . . objective study and planning in many fields. . . . It will require new attitudes, new ways of thinking and acting on the part of the public and the professions." [3]

An approach to such comprehensive planning for elderly persons, including those suffering from prolonged illness, has been made with the enactment of the historic Social Security Amendments of 1965 (Title XVIII) which established a system of health insurance for people over 65 eligible for social security, popularly known as Medicare. This program consists of two parts: Part A provides for a basic program of hospital care, as well as nursing home and home care services following hospitalization and is financed through the social security system. Part B provides for a voluntary prepayment plan by the insured, supplemented by the federal government, to pay for physicians' fees and other services not covered by the basic plan. This part is administered through nonprofit insurance agencies. The significance of this legislation lies not only in the fact that it helps to relieve the elderly

[3] Scheele, p. 49.

of a considerable part of the heavy burden of medical expenses, but that it provides a continuity of care both in the hospital and in the community as well as prescribing standards for such care.

It is unfortunate that till now no such provision had been made for the younger age group afflicted with prolonged illness. This group, as part of the total population faced with heavy medical expenses, can receive aid under Title XIX of the same Amendments, popularly known as Medicaid, if they can prove financial need and if the state in which they live adopts the program.

Despite the limitations of the Medicaid program, the adoption of the 1965 amendments to the social security law points to the emergence of the "new attitudes, new ways of thinking and acting" which the Surgeon General of the U.S. Public Health Service found to be needed.

Recent developments in the field of mental health, better understanding of mental illness and its treatment, hold promise of better care for the chronically mentally sick patient. It is now recognized that in some instances the chronically ill mental patients, who in the past were often forgotten in the back wards of mental hospitals, can be helped through modern methods of treatment, drugs as well as individual and group therapy.

Of particular importance in this connection is the passage of the Community Mental Health Act of 1963. This act made possible the establishment of community-centered mental health centers providing coordinated mental health services, combining inpatient, outpatient, and emergency care, with the patient moving freely from one type of care to another. It is hoped that with the use of such facilities early manifestations of mental illness can be recognized and treated. Also, the movement of patients in and out of the hospital, as their condition requires, should eliminate the fear that hospitalization is the end of the road.

PREVENTION

The adage that "prevention is better than cure" is perhaps nowhere more applicable than in the case of prolonged illness. In the present state of medical knowledge, however, instituting measures which would prevent the development of certain chronic conditions, such as cancer, is unfortunately neither a feasible nor a realistic objective.

The etiology of many of the prolonged illnesses is still unknown. Equally unknown is the influence of the various factors—medical, social, and emotional—which lead to chronicity. Though a beginning has been made in studying some of these factors, research is still confined to all too few institutions. Even given adequate recognition of its importance, such research is at best a slow, time-consuming process requiring a large expenditure of energy and money.

EARLY DETECTION

While the possibility of preventing and curing many of the prolonged illnesses may have to wait for extension of our present medical knowledge, it does not mean that there is nothing that we can do in the meantime. One of the most hopeful advances is the recognition that the earlier control measures are instituted, the greater the likelihood of obviating the progressive, deteriorating, and crippling residual disabilities. The realization that prolonged illness does not appear suddenly in old age but has its beginnings in youth and early adult life points the way to the possible means for discovery of incipient conditions and the prevention of crippling complications. The importance of this recognition is emphasized by the National Health Survey of 1935–36 in this statement: "If the significance of the fact that chronic disease appears at early ages were fully appreciated and more adequate action in the field of public health were taken," there would not be such "an acceleration after the age of

30." [4] This statement remains true today. The same point is emphasized by Dr. E. P. Boas, a recognized authority on the problems of the chronically ill:

The most hopeful aspect of the intensified interest in this problem of chronic diseases is the fact that we have made a turnabout, that we no longer place our chief emphasis on salvaging people in the late stages of these chronic illnesses, but that we are addressing ourselves to an attempt to discover these conditions early, to control their development, and possibly to achieve their prevention.[5]

In our effort to take advantage of whatever available knowledge we possess, we have been handicapped by the failure of the problem to capture the interest of the medical scientist, by the community's acceptance of this lack of interest and concern, and by the resignation so often manifested by the patients themselves. Now that the community has awakened to the threat of prolonged illness for ever larger sections of the population, the pressure of its demand will undoubtedly result in greater and more concentrated effort.

Let us consider some of the actual steps that can be taken in attacking these problems before they reach the stage of chronicity and degeneration. We have learned that in some instances the progress of an existing condition can be controlled. It is true that some of these control measures are not new and have been resorted to as a matter of good common sense for many years. For instance, it has long been recognized that adequate rest, weight control, and reduced exertion are important in lessening the burden on a damaged heart. Similarly, the effect of excitement on blood pressure has been so well appreciated that an excitable person may be frequently admonished, "Watch your blood pressure!" Scientific investigations and our awareness of the interrelation-

[4] U.S. Public Health Service, *The Magnitude of the Chronic Disease Problem in the United States*, p. 10.
[5] Boas, "Clinical Problems," p. 23.

ship between emotional states and physical manifestations lend weight and significance to these common-sense observations. Armed with this understanding, and fortified by the sanction of medical authority, we have a firmer basis on which to build a program of public education. To be fully effective, such a program should include not only instruction in wholesome living, physical as well as mental, but the dissemination of knowledge that in the absence of specific preventive measures, recognition of the importance of early detection, prompt diagnosis, and adequate treatment to arrest the extension of damage constitute our first line of attack.

In this attempt to discover and treat illness in its early stages, the very nature of prolonged illness, with its insidious onset and the transient character or even complete absence of early symptoms, presents a serious obstacle. To overcome it would require a new orientation on the part of the community with emphasis on the need for periodic health examinations as a first step in a program of preventive, diagnostic, and curative medicine. As part of this total program of community education, the general medical practitioner must acquire a greater awareness of, and a conviction of the need for, thorough diagnostic procedures, not only for the evaluation of early symptomatology, but as a routine even in the absence of symptoms. With such a combined attack from the population who are the potential victims of prolonged illness and the medical scientist who is called upon to treat it, some gains can confidently be expected.

The advisability of annual physical examinations has been repeatedly emphasized. Unfortunately, however, the number of people who adhere to a schedule of regular annual check-ups is still small. The time and expense involved, coupled with the natural disinclination of people to go to a doctor when they are symptom-free and experience no discomfort, means that even those who are able to afford them do not take advantage of regular examinations. For large sections of the population, the cost is prohibitive. As a matter of fact, the expenditure of time on the part of the doctor is such an important factor that serious question has been raised as to whether we would have sufficient medical facilities to render such a service to any but a very small portion of the population.

We have seen within our lifetime a concerted effort in several directions aimed at early case-finding. Among these developments, the school health service requirement of a complete physical examination, with provision for follow-up of defects, and the periodic health examinations adopted by some of the industrial organizations represent steps in the right direction. These programs accomplish a double purpose. They are at one and the same time tools for the preservation of health as well as for the early detection and arrest of minor defects which might eventually result in major abnormalities. Unfortunately, all too often the examinations are perfunctory and incomplete, and adequate provision to insure follow-up care is lacking.

Cancer-detection centers.—Among the organizations which serve as media for early case-finding are the cancer-detection centers, which have expanded rapidly. Their primary aim is to alert the population to the need of early cancer diagnosis. The experience of these centers indicates that they have served not only as a means of discovering cancerous and precancerous conditions. In addition, they have detected many correctible pathologies, noncancerous in nature, which might develop into chronic ailments and of which the patients were totally unaware.

An effort to detect early signs of breast cancer not discernable during the ordinary physical examination has been made in a study undertaken by the National Cancer Institute and the Health Insurance Plan of Greater New York (HIP).[6] In this study 30,000 women at the age group par-

---

[6] Sam Shapiro, *et al.*, p. 731.

ticularly susceptible to breast cancer were to be given special mammography (soft tissue x-ray) tests and the results were to be compared with a control group. Preliminary findings indicate that this type of screening "leads to earlier detection of breast cancer than is ordinarily experienced and that mammography contributes significantly to detection." The authors warn that the findings "must be viewed with caution since the study is still in its early stages." A five-year follow-up plan is projected to determine whether mortality from breast cancer can be reduced by this screening method.

Group medical practice.—Another notable advance is the expansion of group medical practice under a plan of voluntary insurance. As was previously pointed out, the proportion of people who carry through on periodic, thorough physical examinations in the absence of specific complaints is small. The frequently prohibitive cost of a complete examination, including special procedures and tests, serves as an additional hindrance. Consequently, we find that unless serious doubt is aroused, physicians often hesitate to press for such complete examinations. Under group medical practice, the question of extra expense for the patient does not enter into consideration. The removal of the cost barrier and the availability of specialists and laboratory facilities mean that all possible diagnostic procedures can be performed, many early indications of possible prolonged illness can be spotted, and immediate treatment instituted. As a result, the objectives of group medical practice "to diagnose accurately; to intervene promptly in diseases or disorders which can be arrested or relieved . . . so that he, the patient, will live as usefully, as happily and as long as his condition and potentialities permit" [7] can be realized.

These and similar efforts illustrate clearly that once a problem is recognized and its importance appreciated, it becomes possible to utilize any number of ways in which it can be attacked. Simultaneously with instituting a wide-

[7] Irving Shapiro, p. 1.

spread system of early case-finding, existing programs can be utilized to assist in the task while performing the duties for which they were originally created. As the necessary skill in detecting early signs of prolonged illness increases, each one of these programs becomes a more and more effective source in early disease diagnosis and treatment. What is even more important, the daily contact with such programs has an influence on the general medical practitioner who, having the opportunity to observe the new concepts at work and convinced of their beneficial results, inevitably carries over some of this thinking into his private practice.

Multiphasic screening.—A new program, known as "multiphasic screening," was inaugurated in 1948. Its major focus was on early case-finding of prolonged illness in unsuspecting victims. One of the early attempts at case-findings through this method was undertaken by Dr. Lester Breslow, who screened over nine hundred industrial workers in California. Since that time, the program has been tried in many communities. It is an attempt to examine "large groups of apparently well people for several diseases at one time, using screening tests only, in order to raise the index of suspicion for the disease for which screening tests have been developed." [8]

According to this definition, multiphasic screening is not intended as a diagnostic procedure. Its objective is to detect incipient signs of unsuspected potential prolonged illness and, if suspicion is aroused, to refer the patient either to his private physician or to medical facilities in the community for more detailed, more specific diagnostic procedures and necessary treatment. It is hoped that by spotting "suspicious" cases the presence of a potential prolonged illness can be detected and early medical care secured, thus improving the prognosis for the patient's future and avoiding some of the tragic intermediate and end results we now see.

Findings confirm the generally prevalent impression that

[8] Chapman, "Multiple Screening—a New Public Health Technique," p. 1.

many victims of prolonged illness are unaware of it. The statement is made that on the basis of the results of tests for seven diseases and checks for significant visual and hearing defects, "tabulations indicate that at least fifty percent of the adult population are affected by chronic disease or chronic physical disabilities of which they are unaware." [9] This is substantiated by an analysis of the first 1,000 cases examined in Boston:

Almost one-half had to be referred to doctors for treatment of un-suspected conditions. The tests uncovered 71 cases of untreated heart disease, 81 of high blood pressure, 48 cases with suspicions of cancer and 21 of diabetes. They also pointed to untreated hearing defects in 63, vision defects in 124, anemia in 16, T.B. in 8, obesity—an insidious shortener of life—in 182, and a variety of other conditions. [In one county in Alabama, it was found that] one in every 12 had heart trouble, diabetes, syphilis, or definite or suspected T.B. [10]

In view of the disastrous effects of prolonged illness on family living and economic productivity, the fact that the majority of those examined were under sixty assumes particular significance.

Among the advantages proclaimed for multiphasic screening are speed of operation and minimal cost to the community. Since the aim is not the establishment of a definite diagnosis, but merely screening for possible signs of disease, the tests can safely be given by technicians, obviating the necessity for employing physicians whose time is valuable and expensive. Another financial saving results from the utilization of available facilities in the particular locality, thus obviating the need for installation of new and expensive setups. In addition, the same tests can be utilized for screening for several diseases. It is first and foremost an important tool in early case-finding of many illnesses whose presence is

[9] Chapman, "Implications and Procedures of Multiphasic Screening," p. 13.
[10] Dublin and Yahres, p. 25.

unsuspected by either the patient or his physician. If suspicious cases are referred immediately and are properly followed up, there is an opportunity to institute treatment early, an important factor in the prevention of disastrous later results.

At the same time, multiphasic screening can serve as a concrete illustration of the need for periodic examinations, even in the absence of actual signs of illness, and in this way can become part of the general scheme of public education. Furthermore, it provides in a limited way a substitute for more extensive periodic health examinations for that part of the population for whom the cost of such examinations is prohibitive. The limited financial resources at their disposal can thus be preserved for diagnostic procedures and treatment, if necessary. As pointed out by Dr. Chapman, "every time a person is found with an early case of chronic illness or chronic disability, treatment can be instituted while that person is still able to earn a living and pay his own bills." [11] As is well known, once an illness has progressed to the stage of chronicity and invalidism, the burden of the cost of medical care is beyond the available resources of most families and has to be borne by the community.

While the soundness of the basic concepts underlying multiphasic screening is undisputed, critics point out that in some instances, owing to the limitations of our present-day scientific knowledge, simple, specific tests are entirely lacking; in others, the tests are not sufficiently sensitive or the levels which indicate pathology not fully determined. Consequently, the results show some "false positives"; that is, patients who do not in reality have a specific disease, are considered "suspicious" and are referred for diagnosis and treatment, while "false negatives," patients who have the disease, are overlooked. The main purpose of early detection is to assure prompt treatment. The most serious drawback

[11] Chapman, "Multiple Screening—a New Public Health Technique," p. 11.

inherent in multiphasic screening is the fact that many of the patients screened as "positive" have actually failed to follow the recommendations to report for further diagnosis and treatment. If we are to measure the effectiveness of multiphasic screening in securing early diagnosis and treatment, we need to devise a system of reporting that indicates the proportion of patients who follow the recommendation for further diagnostic procedures. We also need to know how many of the patients who required treatment actually received it. Such a system of reporting would have to be sufficiently simple to insure its being followed by physicians and outpatient departments, and sufficiently comprehensive to make it valuable.

The importance of follow-up of conditions found through a screening process is being tested in a special screening program conducted by the Permanent Medical Group of Oakland, California. In this program the appointment for the screening examination is made by the person's physician, who is immediately informed of the findings. It is hoped that as a result of this close connection between the physician and the screening center there will be a higher probability of follow-up. Similarly, in the study of examinations for breast cancer previously discussed, the results of the screening process are available to the patient's physician.

Because of the large number of cases where patients did not follow up the results of the screening process, reliance is put more and more frequently on the preventive measures for specific diseases. For instance, in the case of cardiac difficulties, studies are concerned with the effects of smoking and the importance of weight control and physical activity as well as with the effects of hypertension.

NEED FOR INTEGRATED PLANNING

Without attempting to minimize the importance of early detection as a first step in a control program, it goes without saying that even the best possible method of case-finding will fall short of its objective unless community facilities are available for further diagnostic study when indicated and for treatment when found necessary. The problem of providing adequate treatment is a problem not only of available or even potential facilities, but of the stage of development of our medical knowledge as well.

While waiting for research and the miracles of science to bring us cures, we must turn our efforts to improving existing community resources for the care of the large number of patients with prolonged illnesses who require attention today, and those who will need it tomorrow. Admittedly, present-day provisions are insufficient in number and inadequate in the type of care given. Our understanding of the varying phases of prolonged illness, coupled with our increased understanding of its psychological implications, supplies the necessary framework for planning the facilities of the future. Just as we found that the doctor alone cannot meet the manifold problems prolonged illness creates, so we now find that no one institution or group of institutions can furnish the total answer for a goup of illnesses so varied in the demands they make upon the patient and the community. Facilities for care will need to be planned, not as isolated entities to provide for the various stages of the illness, but as an integrated whole, if we are to assure for the patients the optimum of medical care and of physical, social, and emotional well-being.

Because of the complexity of the problem, it will help if future planning is geared to meeting the problems presented by the four-stage process of prolonged illness referred to earlier. Each stage determines the patient's capacity to cope, unaided, with the problems he faces, the amount and kind of help he will need from others, and consequently the type of facilities most adapted for effective medical care.

HOSPITAL FACILITIES OF THE FUTURE

Let us begin with the patient who needs active medical treatment in a hospital. It is at this point that the severity of the problem is most acute, the patient almost completely incapacitated and, at the same time, subjected to the greatest physical and emotional strain. As our previous discussion indicated, little has been done so to gear our treatment as to encompass all the facets of the problem these patients present, or to integrate our broader understanding of the social problems involved wih the medical treatment. The amount of care provided is woefully insufficient, not only qualitatively, but even quantitatively. We hear a great deal about the inadequate number of hospital beds. Do we really know how many are needed for the care of patients with prolonged illness?

So far, we have no accurate count of patients with prolonged illness, nor does it seem possible to arrive at an accurate count under existing conditions. The nearest approximation is given in the U.S. Public Health Study on Chronic Conditions and Activity Limitations. However, the number of 80.3 million persons with chronic conditions, estimated by that study, is admittedly low since it does not include those persons who were in institutions at the time, nor those who were chronically ill mentally.

In the absence of systematic planning, patients and their families, when no longer able to cope with the problem unaided, have sought refuge wherever they could. Under these conditions, the place of refuge had little if any relation to the patient's actual condition or the type of care he required. It is reasonable to assume that if we were to make a survey of the present population afflicted with prolonged illness, we would probably find many patients languishing in custodial institutions who would be happier and better off living in the community, provided the community were geared to meeting their needs. On the other hand, we would be just as likely to find patients in their homes who could profit by being in a hospital where they would have the advantages of intensive medical treatment which would prepare them for eventual functioning in the community. Similarly, among the patients cared for in their homes we would undoubtedly find a number who present unbearable burdens to their families and should be in custodial institutions.

The situation as it affects the care of patients with prolonged illness was described graphically by Dr. E. P. Boas in 1940, and his statement still holds true:

The existing facilities for the care of the chronic sick present a very confused picture . . . patients at home who should be in hospitals, patients in homes for the aged that are not prepared to minister to their wants, patients in convalescent homes occupying beds needed for another purpose, a mad confusion of patients and institutions—the patients scrambling to find refuge wherever they may, the institutions admitting them grudgingly, and having admitted them, not providing the care that they need. It is a scene of great disorder . . . public and private hospitals, homes for the aged, convalescent homes, nursing and visiting doctor services, aftercare agencies, agencies for sheltered work, medical social service departments, family service agencies—everyone of them accepts with reluctance the burden of the chronic sick, and tries to shift responsibility to another agency which is no better prepared for the task.[12]

Actual findings based on carefully conducted studies substantiate these general statements made on the basis of observation and wide experience. For instance, in a study conducted by the Community Council of Greater New York to determine the adequacy of facilities for the care of patients incapacitated by prolonged illness, it was found that in New York City custodial homes and homes for the aged have many

[12] Boas, *The Unseen Plague: Chronic Diseases*, p. 75.

patients needing hospital care, and hospital beds are occupied by patients requiring only custodial care.[13]

A study conducted by the U. S. Public Health Service as late as 1963 confirms these earlier findings. An analysis of the physical status of the residents of nursing and personal care homes leaves no doubt that many of them suffer from prolonged illness. On the other hand, the study mentions that "nursing and personal care to the aged and chronically ill is also provided in chronic disease hospitals as well as nursing home units and chronic disease wards of general hospitals." [14]

The net result of all this confusion is detrimental to the patient, who frequently does not receive the care he requires when he needs it, who is shifted from one place to another, and who, in the process, loses whatever sense of security and faith he may still have in the ability of medical science to help him and in his own capacity to recover.

It might well be that what is needed as much as additional hospital facilities is a redistribution of available facilities in accordance with our better understanding of the requirements of the patient.

If future planning for the patient with prolonged illness is to meet his needs more adequately than hitherto, it must be based on our current thinking about the problems he presents and our understanding of the best way to meet these problems. In the past the planning was based on the prevailing feeling of hopelessness in handling "chronic" patients and was therefore primarily concerned with providing institutional care for people in the advanced stages of disease.

What, then, happens to the patient in need of hospital care and treatment? We find that the exigencies of the reality situation break down the artificial barriers between "acute"

[13] Jarrett, p. 22.
[14] U.S. Public Health Service, *Characteristics of Residents in Institutions for the Aged and Chronically Ill*, p. 10.

and "chronic," and the patient with prolonged illness is usually admitted to the "acute" general hospital when an acute exacerbation of his illness makes hospitalization imperative. Unfortunately, however, the "acute" general hospital admits these patients grudgingly, and only when forced to do so by the acuteness of the immediate episode. Feeling that the patient does not belong there, the hospital often insists upon his leaving before he is ready for discharge. Usually there is pressure both on the part of the hospital administration and of the medical staff for his removal, even though they are aware that facilities for adequate care elsewhere are lacking. While the reason most frequently given is the urgent need of beds for the more acutely ill patients, other factors unquestionably influence the decision. The paucity of scientific knowledge about prolonged illness and the consequent hopelessness with which the patient is still regarded, the feeling of helplessness and failure he engenders in the physician, the absence of medical urgency and dramatic appeal—all these contribute to the fact that such a patient is not wanted in the general hospital. In the absence of adequate facilities for continued medical care, the patient is sent either to his home, with little if any provision for further medical care, or, if a bed can be secured, to a public "home" with lower standards, where the care is largely of a custodial nature. Such care is too often totally inadequate to meet his needs or to provide continued treatment which would insure the maintenance of whatever benefits he might have derived from his hospitalization.

The recognition of all these difficulties imposes an obligation to find ways to care for the evergrowing number of patients with prolonged illness. This will require a change in our thinking about such patients and their needs, as well as an over-all planning based not merely on the need to meet an emergency situation, but on a long-range point of view. It implies first and foremost a modification of society's attitude that prolonged illness is hopeless and that therefore the expense of intensive medical care would be unjustified, useless, and wasted. It means the abandonment of our previous inclination to consider such patients as separate and different, not amenable to medical treatment, easily expendable. Above all, it means our assuming the responsibility of planning for them as an integral part of the total community planning for medical and health services.

It is indeed a hopeful sign that the plans being proposed by those with knowledge of, and interest in, prolonged illness indicate an understanding of the nature of the problem and, consequently, a better integration of all facilities with the hope that such an integration would provide more adequate care and bring about better results in treatment, without necessarily involving larger financial outlays for the community. Taking into consideration the changes to be expected in the physical condition of the patient afflicted with prolonged illness, changes which require different types of medical attention at different periods, these plans are more closely attuned to the patient's actual needs at the moment and are not based on the artificial separation created by the concepts of "acuteness" or "chronicity." In line with this point of view it becomes evident that no patient who requires hospital care should be denied admission on the basis of diagnosis or be forced to leave the hospital merely because of an arbitrary time limit, but should remain as long as his medical condition requires hospital care.

As a preliminary for planning adequate facilities, it is essential to have some estimate of the number of patients in need of hospitalization. For a long time we have been handicapped by the absence of reliable information about the actual extent of prolonged illness or probable future trends.

In 1938 a survey was published covering all the facilities available for the care of the sick in New York City and the metropolitan area. On the basis of this survey the recommendation was made for the establishment of a "permanent, representative and authoritative" community agency to plan and coordinate hospital facilities and services in New York City.[15] As a result of these recommendations, the Hospital Council of Greater New York published the Master Plan for Hospitals and Related Facilities for New York City and recommended "that there be three types of general care hospitals—community, regional, and central. . . . As stated in the constitution, the Hospital Council proceeded to plan the efficient and economical development of hospitals and other facilities for the care of the sick serving New York City in accordance with measured needs for these services and available resources." [16]

Recognizing that the hospital needs and hospital services in New York City and the suburbs are closely related, the responsibilities of the Hospital Council of Greater New York were extended to embrace both the city and the suburbs. In 1961 it became the Hospital Review and Planning Council of Southern New York.

Within this plan, the needs of the patients with prolonged illness receive individual and careful attention as an important part of such a program. In accord with our most up-to-date thinking, the study takes into consideration not only the needs of the community for medical facilities, but also the needs of the hospitals in providing teaching and training as well as research facilities for the professional personnel, so that they may be better equipped to render the necessary medical care. It was the opinion of the Council, however, that the principles of the plan could be adapted to apply beyond that period, in line with changing conditions. The provisions to meet the estimated needs were intended for all economic strata, thus giving recognition to the fact that the

[15] The Hospital Council of Greater New York, p. 1.
[16] Annual Report of the Hospital Council of Greater New York, 1959–60, p. 9.

need for, as well as the inadequacy of, facilities holds true for the rich as well as the poor.

It was the recommendation of the Hospital Council that hospitals for patients with prolonged illness who require active medical treatment should be provided as units of general hospitals and not separate institutions. In this the Hospital Council was supported by all known authorities in the field. As far back as 1944 Dr. E. M. Bluestone expressed the opinion that "the establishment of independent hospitals for chronic disease of whatever designation, at a distance and at comparatively greater expense if the job is to be done right, should be discouraged." [17] Subsequent developments have fully justified this contention.

There is at present a fairly consistent agreement that separate hospitals for the care of patients with prolonged illness, even if possible, would be inadvisable. It is argued that combined facilities would eliminate many undesirable features of the existing facilities. Close physical proximity of facilities for "acute" and "chronic" patients would eliminate the discrimination against the latter group now practiced by many of the general hospitals, would result in better care for the different phases of prolonged illness, would assure ease of transfer in accordance with the demands of the patient's medical condition, and would obviate the duplication of expensive facilities. In addition, such proximity would provide opportunity and incentive for interest in study and research into the causes and nature of prolonged illness. Finally, since prolonged illness is so often the sequel of an acute episode, the medical practitoner would have an opportunity to observe the end results of his treatment of acute conditions and hopefully to learn from such observation.

NURSING HOMES AS PART OF TOTAL MEDICAL CARE

While some patients with prolonged illness require active medical care in a hospital or at home for lengthy periods and

[17] Bluestone, "The Chronic Has a Claim," p. 68.

others may need permanent custodial placement, such illness does not necessarily imply either permanent incapacity or lifelong invalidism. As medical science advances and new methods of treatment are discoverd, more and more patients, having emerged from an acute episode, can proceed on the way to a normal or near-normal resumption of activity. Like many of the acutely ill patients, however, they may require a period of convalescence to help with the gradual transition from the sheltered environment of the hospital to normal living in the community.

As the importance of the convalescence has become more widely recognized, there has developed a growing understanding of the need for closer integration between the medical institution where active treatment is being given and an institution which would insure the continuity of medical, nursing, and dietetic supervision which many of these patients require. Some authorities claim that the availability of convalescent wards would drastically reduce the number of readmissions to the more expensive hospital facilities. The latter would then become more readily available for those patients who urgently need them.

The inadequacy of existing facilities can be readily understood if we keep in mind that they just grew, springing up in response to particular pressures from time to time. Because of the general lack of interest in prolonged illness, no concerted effort was made in the past either to integrate them into one comprehensive whole or to improve their individual functioning. Future planning presupposes a different approach based on a better understanding on the part of the community, and the convalescent home, of the medical-social needs of the convalescent patient.

If this is to be achieved, the entire orientation of the community, the medical profession, and the convalescent home will have to be changed. Convalescence can no longer be regarded as merely a rest or a vacation, nor can a place be classified as a convalescent home simply because it is located in country surroundings. The convalescent facilities of the future, whether they be located on hospital grounds or at a distance, will have to remain under the medical supervision of the hospital. If it is to fulfill its part in the restoration of the patient to maximal usefulness, the convalescent period will have to be utilized constructively and dynamically as part of a well-rounded medical-social program.

Since convalescence comes at a time when the urgency of the medical problem recedes into the background, this period can be utilized to focus attention more effectively on the patient's social, familial, and emotional problems. Help may be needed in three main areas. The patient's environment may require modification to meet his individual needs. Family members may need help to insure their acceptance of the patient and to enlist their cooperation in regaining a place for him in the life of the family and the community. Most important of all, the patient himself may profitably use help in preparing for a return to normal living.

A period of convalescence provides the necessary opportunity for weaning the patient from the dependency engendered by the illness and for guiding him toward more mature living in the community. For it is at this time that the patient's interest, centered primarily upon himself during illness, is directed to the world outside—his family, friends, work, community affairs. As his normal goals begin to reassert themselves once again, he will need help if he is to adjust them to whatever limitations the residue of the illness imposes upon him. In addition, if the gains achieved during hospitalization are to be preserved, the convalescence can be utilized to instill rules of health, to initiate the practice of preventive medicine, and to teach the patient that the maintenance of maximal physical well-being is part of the broader goal for a fuller and richer life.

All these aspects of help to the patient and to his family are essential if the ultimate goal of comprehensive medical care —restoration of the patient to normal and healthful living within the community—is to be brought to a successful conclusion.

The goal of gradual convalescence under medical, nursing, and dietetic supervision is envisioned in the provision of nursing home care in the federal Medicare program. Under this program, nursing homes are considered to be extended care facilities to be affiliated with one or more hospitals in close proximity to facilitate transfer of patients when such transfer is authorized by the hospital physician.

The Medicare program sets high standards for nursing homes. It requires continued medical supervision, skilled nursing care, the maintenance of adequate records, the establishment of policies governing services rendered, and the review of such services by a professional group which must include at least one physician and one nurse. Social service evaluation of home conditions as well as the patient's needs and referral for such services as may be indicated is also required. It is estimated that less than one third of all nursing homes now in operation will qualify for Medicare recognition under these requirements. To help alleviate the shortage, the U.S. Public Health Service through the Hill-Burton Act makes grants available to state and local governments and to nonprofit organizations for "the construction, expansion, alteration and remodeling of nursing homes." [18]

IMPROVEMENT OF CUSTODIAL FACILITIES

As was indicated earlier, indiscriminate planning in the past has resulted not only in an inadequate number of beds for patients with prolonged illness, but in an improper use of existing facilities as well. While on the one hand there are not enough beds to care for patients who need active medical treatment, on the other, hospital beds are occupied by patients

[18] President's Council on Aging, "Federal Aid for Nursing Homes," p. 3.

who no longer require such care. Admittedly, those patients whose disease is stationary or very slowly progressive are in need not of hospital but of custodial care. They are often kept in the hospital merely because of lack of other institutional facilities.

As we survey the custodial institutions, we cannot fail to be impressed by their inadequacies. As was indicated earlier in this book, whether conducted under public or private auspices they too often fail to meet the existing need both quantitatively and qualitatively. And yet, our present-day concept of prolonged illness views the custodial institution as an essential facility for care in certain of its phases, provided that the patient is ineligible for hospitalization and has no home.

Any program of total medical care would, of necessity, have to make adequate provision for the patients requiring it. There can be but little question that more facilities, both public and private, will need to be built. Numbers alone will not meet the problem, however. A concerted effort will have to be made to insure a more adequate type of care. This would include the establishment of standards covering physical facilities as well as the number and qualifications of personnel, the amount and kind of medical and nursing supervision, and the provision of such other services as would enable patients to lead as full and as satisfying a life as their condition permits. It goes without saying that such standards would be useless unless there were machinery to guarantee their enforcement.

Location of the custodial institution not too far from the life of the community is another essential prerequisite. Adequate medical supervision through integration with a medical institution, so that a patient may be easily hospitalized should the need arise, is still another.

Integration of the custodial institution in total planning for the care of the patient, attention to its location, and continued medical supervision would help to eliminate some of the hopelessness which prolonged illness connotes at present. It would mean, among other things, that the transfer of a patient to a custodial institution would not necessarily imply his consignment to oblivion. The continued interest of a medical institution and the rendering of adequate medical help would demonstrate that the welfare of the patient continues to be a matter of concern to those who have assumed responsibility for his total medical care.

Important as institutional facilities may be, whether for active medical treatment or custodial care, they are not the only answer for patients suffering from prolonged illness. Many of these patients, who no longer need specialized and concentrated hospital facilities but who still require intensive medical and nursing supervision, can be cared for in their own homes. The pioneering home care program at Montefiore Hospital and the subsequent home care programs of the city hospitals in New York have shown that care in the home is not only an acceptable substitute to relieve the shortage of hospital beds, but may actually prove to be the better choice so far as the patient is concerned, providing individualization of care, as envisioned by the author of the program. After twenty years of operation, Montefiore's home care program has amply proved that given careful selection of patients and adequate medical and social supervision, the care these patients receive can be maintained on a level equal to that in the hospital, while the numerous problems inherent in prolonged hospitalization, removal from accustomed surroundings, and all the other problems which have been discussed in detail earlier in this book, can be eliminated.

When the program was originally organized at Montefiore, it was thought that its ultimate usefulness would be determined by the extent to which it would remain flexible enough to allow for adaptation to individual differences in the patients and families to be served as well as to the requirements of the setting in which it would operate. The value of flexibility was subsequently proved as other hospitals instituted similar programs suited to their particular requirements.

The concept of home care as part of a comprehensive plan of medical care which was included in the Medicare program for patients at home following hospitalization is testimony to the original philosophy underlying the so-called "traditional Montefiore home care program," namely, that it is a means of providing better care for patients while, at the same time, freeing badly needed hospital beds.

An additional demonstration of the usefulness of home care in the total treatment plan for patients is its recent adoption for patients covered by hospital insurance through Blue Cross. As the character of the hospital population changed and the number of insured patients increased, the Associated Hospital Service of New York (AHS), popularly known as Blue Cross, entered into agreement with a number of voluntary accredited hospitals and public health nursing agencies to offer a modified form of home care to patients covered by its insurance.

Plans for the patient's transfer home are made by the physician, the patient, a member of his family, and the nurse coordinator, taking into consideration the patient's medical, nursing, and social needs. While he is on the AHS home care program the patient remains under the care of his private physician, with nursing service provided through the community nursing agency. Other services which would have been made available in the hospital are provided, within practical limits, by or through the hospital.

According to the AHS reports, the home care experience has demonstrated its advantages to the satisfaction of physicians, patients, and families. At the same time, the program serves to reduce the cost of care for both the patient and the AHS. Thus the AHS annual report, dated June, 1962, states:

"The experience of the Associated Hospital Service in providing home care to semi-private patients has demonstrated that the cost of the combined hospital stay and home care is about 25% less than the total payment which had been made for hospital care alone." [19] At the same time, it enables the patient to conserve the number of days of hospitalization to which he is entitled under his contract.

The expansion of home care programs and their importance for the welfare of the patient led to the establishment of special training centers for which training grants were made available through the U.S. Public Health Service. Three of these centers were established in hospital-based home care programs—Montefiore Hospital among them—and in one community-based home care program. These training centers provide intensive supervised clinical experience in the team management and bedside care of homebound chronically ill patients. The course consists of educational programs as well as field training and deals with the philosophy and history of home care, criteria for selection, structural patterns and trends. It is open to administrative and operational personnel who are involved in organizing and operating home care programs.

An evaluation of home care treatment of prolonged illness points up its important contribution in demonstrating the effectiveness of the multidiscipline approach. Seeing the patient in his own home emphasizes that the illness, disabling as it might be, does not rob him of his place as a person in the family and in the community, or of his dignity as a human being and his right to live as full a life as he can as long as he lives.

We may reasonably question whether we have been overzealous in our attempts to "sell" the hospital as the only place, or at least the first place of choice, for the care of the sick. It is true that certain diagnostic procedures and certain

[19] Associated Hospital Service, p. 33.

medical and surgical treatments can best be performed in a hospital. Home care programs have shown, however, that many phases of treatment, which until now were thought to be possible only in a hospital setting, can be carried out just as effectively in the home. It has also been proved beyond any shadow of doubt that patients react favorably to being away from an institutional environment, close to family and friends, and being able to lead a more nearly normal existence as they participate in family living. Even the fact that they are able to sleep in their own beds and have home-cooked meals assumes significance and adds to their contentment. With the background of understanding of the inter-relation of mental and physical components in illness, it is not surprising that in many instances this sense of well-being has been reflected in a better response to medical treatment and thus in actual physical improvement. Since our concern is with the total welfare of the patient, this fact is of the utmost importance in considering the inclusion of home care programs in any over-all planning.

From a practical point of view, the high cost of building and maintaining hospitals means that indefinite expansion of such facilities, even were it advisable, would be prohibitive; a staggering burden for the community to carry. Any planning for meeting future needs would, therefore, be better planning if extension of home care were given the attention it deserves, since it provides the necessary care at a fraction of hospital cost. To quote the still cogent words of the master plan: "The cost for hospital care is steadily increasing to the point where it becomes necessary to provide as much care as possible during the ambulatory period. Provision of home care and extension of home nursing service . . . should materially reduce the number of patients who must be admitted to the hospital." [20] The economy of a home care program thus becomes an additional argument for the exten-

[20] The Hospital Council of Greater New York, p. 36.

sion of home care facilities for suitable patients and under careful safeguards.

Following a period of convalescence and readjustment, many patients can return to functioning within the community. The very nature of the illness, however, and the ever present threat of an acute exacerbation of symptoms often necessitate continued medical supervision and follow-up, which can be secured on an outpatient basis. What has been said about other facilities for the care of the patient with prolonged illness applies with equal force to the care in hospital clinics and outpatient departments: they are inadequate both in number and in the care they provide. Our planning in this, as in other areas, must take into consideration not only their shortcomings in relation to the patients who now need their services, but even more their inadequacy for the care of the growing number of patients who will require this service in the years to come. If clinic visits are to accomplish their purpose, namely, to maintain the gains secured through hospitalization and to spot and treat early manifestations of relapse, the spread of the disease, or concurrent illnesses, more precise and individualized attention is essential to replace the present-day perfunctory examination and the admonition to "return in two weeks."

It will be necessary to integrate attendance at the clinic with the total plan for medical care. With due attention to the patient as a person, clinic attendance could then be utilized to promote his welfare—social and emotional as well as physical; for in addition to the medical follow-up, the outpatient department holds other values for the patient. Frequently, it represents his only source of social contact in an otherwise restricted life. Long periods in the hospital encourage the formation of friendships based on similar experiences and similar problems. Attendance at the clinic gives the patient an opportunity to continue these friendships. The very contact with similarly handicapped individuals counteracts to some extent the feeling of difference that he feels so strongly in the world outside. It would seem that until now little advantage has been taken of the waiting periods at clinics and the yearning that these patients show for social contacts.

An article in *Lancet,* reporting on an experiment conducted at the Latilla Physiotherapy Department at the Royal Sussex County Hospital, Brighton, England, points out that "a great deal of the benefit they [the patients] derived from attendance as out-patients was from human fellowship rather than from the ritual medical advice and bottle of physic." A club was organized to give the patients an opportunity for social contacts, and the author reports that the patients "look forward to the meetings which 'make a break' and are 'jolly good treatment.' " The author states that "hospitals should accept, as part of their function, the duty to re-able and encourage these patients through social activities" and concludes that the principle is "to pick from the population of out-patient departments the crippled, lonely and aging and help to keep them mobile, active and purposeful, to find them friends, and to show them they are not peculiar, isolated cases and that other people who are equally handicapped can do things, be real persons, and find life worth while." [21]

In an effort to overcome the depressing features of the clinic waiting rooms, several hospitals have organized recreational activities both for inpatients and outpatients. All those concerned in the experiment agree that such a program tends to dispel tension and nervousness and takes away from the dreariness and depressing atmosphere of the waiting room.

Anyone familiar with the atmosphere of a clinic waiting room, with its rows of benches occupied by the ailing, the

[21] Bourne, p. 127.

crippled, the disabled and disfigured, will welcome any program which brings cheer and relief from tension. Since it appears that it is difficult, if not impossible, to shorten the waiting periods, much more could be done to build an extended program which would make the most of the possibilities inherent in clinical visits. With a better understanding of what clinic contacts can mean to patients, and the development of an appreciation of the value of group interaction, the waiting time could be constructively utilized to provide not only recreation, but a rehabilitation program through occupational facilities and therapeutic group discussions with skilled leadership.

OUTLINE OF A COMPREHENSIVE
PROGRAM OF CARE

These, then, are the existing facilities for the care of patients with prolonged illness. Having pointed up their inadequacies and having suggested what changes must be made if the future care of these patients is to be in line with our heightened understanding of the illness, let us review briefly the plan here outlined.

We can envision a network of integrated facilities, with the medical institution as the center, for the primary purpose of providing as adequate and well-rounded care as possible for the sick person, whether his illness be "acute" or "chronic." The actual setting, whether a hospital, his home, or some intermediary institution, would be determined not by traditional, artificial lines of demarcation, but by the patient's medical needs at any particular time with provision for free movement from one place of care to another, depending upon the changing demands of his medical condition.

Under such a plan patients with prolonged illness requiring hospitalization would be cared for in wings of, or in buildings attached to, a general hospital. Admission to a hospital would be governed by the patient's need for a hospital bed, because he needed intensive medical supervision, a thorough laboratory work-up, major surgery, or the use of heavy equipment.[22] All facilities for treatment, study, and research would be available to such patients in the same way as they are now available to the acutely ill, with provision for such additional equipment as some of the prolonged illnesses require. With the acceptance of the premise that a sick person has a right to a hospital bed as long as he requires the use of hospital facilities, the length of stay would be determined solely by his medical condition and not by arbitrarily set time limits.

No patient would occupy a hospital bed when he was no longer able to profit from specialized hospital facilities. His discharge, however, would not mean merely a decision "to get rid of him." Recognizing that hospitalization is but one step in the treatment of prolonged illness, the hospital would continue the responsibility it assumed at the time of admission, by making arrangements for the type of care needed by the particular patient at the particular time. Planning for total medical care would be based on the philosophy that the responsibility for medical care and supervision cannot be laid aside at any particular point but must be continued as long as the need exists. In the case of the patient with prolonged illness, this responsibility may last as long as the patient lives.

The patient who could be treated on an outpatient basis would be referred to his own physician, if he were able to carry the financial burden this would impose; if he could not finance private care, he would be referred to the outpatient department of a hospital.

If no longer in need of hospital care and treatment, but unable to function on an outpatient basis or to meet the fees charged by a private physician, the patient would be cared for in his own home, or a substitute home, with the hospital

[22] Bluestone. "Medical Care for Patients with Prolonged Illness," p. 149.

assuming responsibility for full medical, nursing, and social service treatment as now practiced under the home care program.

The patient no longer requiring active medical treatment, but in need of a period of recuperation following hospitalization, would be transferred to a convalescent institution closely affiliated with a hospital, thus assuring continuity of medical supervision and the provision of rehabilitative services as a preparation for return to community living.

Custodial care would be available for the patient with residual illness who could not be cared for at home. Our increased appreciation of the needs of the custodial patient would no longer allow us to be satisfied with poor farms or almshouses away from centers of treatment and research. The custodial institution would afford continuity of medical supervision through a tie-up with a medical institution and the opportunity for free transfer to a hospital should the patient's condition require it. In addition, recognition would be given to the fact that the patient has needs other than those arising from the demands of his illness. Consequently, in addition to maintaining acceptable standards of physical comfort and adequate nursing care, the custodial institution would make provision for occupational and recreational therapy. The location of the institution would be given careful consideration, for it would be recognized that it must be accessible to friends and relatives if the patient is not to feel abandoned and forgotten.

NEED FOR ATTENTION TO SOCIAL AND EMOTIONAL FACTORS

The concept of an over-all program of medical care here discussed does more than make provision for a continuity of expert medical care of the highest level. It would insure integrated treatment of the patient's medical, social, and emotional needs. It shifts the focus of attention from treatment of the illness to treatment of the patient.

It is recognized that in prolonged illness emotional factors are of etiological, diagnostic, and therapeutic significance.[23] If our attempts to ameliorate the disastrous aftereffects of prolonged illness are not to be in vain, we will need further inquiry into, and a better understanding of, the interaction of physical, social, and emotional factors in illness. The integration of all medical facilities, with the hospital as the center, would offer a rich opportunity for continuity of research into causes and sequelae of prolonged illness, into the interrelation between medical, social, and emotional problems and methods of scientific attack upon such illness in all its phases.

As we learn the specific ways in which these interrelationships manifest themselves, the medical team caring for the patient will gradually develop a new orientation and a willingness to consider these nonmedical factors in the plan of treatment. Such an approach will help, among other things, to eliminate some of the hopelessness now associated with prolonged illness; for we will no longer be inclined to throw up our hands in despair merely because we are not able to alter the unrelenting progress of the disease. Instead, it will enable us to see that no matter how far the disease has progressed, no matter how incapacitated the patient, he remains a living human being with needs which we must make an effort to satisfy. The medical practitioner who, in his daily contact with the sick person, has the opportunity to observe the interrelationship between the patient's emotional needs and his physical well-being has an important contribution to make. It is to him that we must look for guidance in the development of a different approach and an enlightened point of view in the care of the sick.

THE FAMILY AS A UNIT OF TREATMENT

Developments in the practice of medicine direct attention to the need to consider the problem of the patient in relation to his total situation if he is to derive all the benefits possible

[23] Getting, p. 1251.

from his medical care. In this concept is included not only the patient's illness and his reaction to it, but his feelings about his family and friends. We have learned long ago that it is impossible to separate the diseased organ from the person to whom it belongs. Nor can we separate the person from the world in which he lives and which fashions and sustains him.

A demonstration project, known as Family Health Maintenance, was inaugurated in 1953, sponsored jointly by the Community Service Society, the College of Physicians and Surgeons of Columbia University, and Montefiore Hospital. The need to concentrate on the preservation of health, emotional as well as physical, grew out of the experience of the Community Service Society in dealing with the individual difficulties and family disintegration that frequently result from illness or disability which might have been prevented. The program, as outlined, was based on the recognition that "health care as at present practiced, even if of high scientific quality, falls short of its potentialities because of inadequate recognition of the psychological and social aspects of such care." [24] We have been wont to think of medical care only as a means to cure or arrest a disease process. By contrast, the Family Health Maintenance demonstration was seen as a means to "improve the health care of families and individuals through placing major emphasis on the maintenance of health and the prevention of unnecessary illness," and to "substitute the concept of health maintenance of positive health for the more prevalent concept of sickness care as a major objective." [25]

Important as were the preventive aspects of this program, its most outstanding contribution was in shifting the focus of attention in medical care from the individual to the family as a unit. It recognized that the family as the basic unit of our

[24] Bluestone, "Social Medicine Arrives in the Hospital," p. 61.
[25] Ibid.

society is also the unit of health and should, therefore, be the unit of treatment.

REHABILITATION NEEDS OF THE FUTURE

In discussing the problems that confront sick people, the question of providing immediate medical care for the illness which brings them to the hospital necessarily assumes major significance and requires primary consideration. The scientific challenge, inherent in combating disease, combined with the medical practitioner's humane desire to arrest suffering and postpone a fatal outcome, has in the past conspired to blind him to the problems these patients are called upon to face once the medical urgency has been met. And yet, all disabled individuals face problems as they attempt to adjust their impaired capacities to the demands of everyday living.

We now recognize that medical science, in arresting the disease process and enabling people to live longer with their handicap, has at the same time assumed the obligation to insure for them as full and rich a life as their condition permits. By making the disabled individual socially useful, by enabling him to engage in such activities as he is capable of undertaking, and by utilizing whatever skills he possesses we can help to minimize his social problems, maintain his morale, and instill in him a feeling of independence and security.

This emphasis has changed the outlook for many patients suffering from severe and irreversible disability which precludes their return to economic productivity. They need no longer feel that they are condemned to a life of complete helplessness, uselessness, and dependence. Whether the aim be adjusting to, compensating for, or overcoming of, the handicap, rehabilitation goals can be set to meet the needs of the individual patient at the particular time, and then advanced in accord with his increasing ability. Whatever the ultimate goal, so far as the patient is concerned, rehabilitation is first and foremost a definite step toward giving up the dependence engendered by illness and hospitalization. From this point of view, even such an infinitesimal gain as being helped to ambulate after a long period of bedridden existence is a beginning in the process of rehabilitation. Every succeeding effort which the patient can make brings him closer to the ultimate he can achieve.

In this process of gradual achievement the patient's personal reaction to his handicap and to the way in which it may change his appearance, restrict his activities, affect his plans for the future, and change his entire mode of living, necessarily comes to the fore. Any change which has such far-reaching implications requires for its eventual success a gradual process of preparation. Rehabilitation plans must, therefore, be instituted early, preferably as soon after the patient's admission to the hospital as his condition permits. In fact, the very initiation of medical care with its emphasis on diagnosis and treatment is the first step in the rehabilitation process.

As pointed out by the Commission on Chronic Illness:

Rehabilitation is an innate element of adequate care and properly begins with diagnosis. It is applicable alike to persons who may become employable and to those whose only realistic hope may be a higher level of self-care. Not only must formal rehabilitation services be supplied as needed, but programs, institutions, and personnel must be aggressively rehabilitation-minded.[26]

Such an early beginning not only provides sufficient time for careful planning, but, even more important, it gives the patient the feeling that he has a future to look forward to, bolsters his hopes, and minimizes his fears. Rehabilitation thus becomes not only the ultimate goal of medical care, but one of the tools at our disposal for the satisfaction of the patient's inner needs.

[26] "The Commission Adopts Further Recommendations on the Care of the Long-Term Patient," p. 1.

The importance of this broadened concept of rehabilitation is evident in the newly awakened interest in the rehabilitation of the aged, a group for whom the goal of return to useful, gainful employment can hardly be envisioned. The fact that a geriatric rehabilitation service has been established at the Goldwater Memorial Hospital on Welfare Island, New York, is one of vast significance; for it recognizes that "no one can stay the passing of years but much can be done to prevent needless suffering and the loss of function and dignity in the older person." [27]

Despite this shift in emphasis, despite our understanding of the need to adjust our goals to the reality limitations imposed by the patient's illness, despite our recognition of the need for such a program, community facilities for this type of service remain inadequate. Neither the extensive program set up for returned servicemen after the First World War nor the utilization of the dynamic forces inherent in group living with others similarly handicapped has as yet been duplicated in the meager services available for the general population. The reasoning most frequently advanced for the difference of approach is the fact that the disabled serviceman is a young man with many years of potentially useful life ahead of him, whereas the patient with prolonged illness is "old and decrepit." This attitude is the result of the prevailing feeling that expensive rehabilitation services should bring tangible economic returns and ignores the values inherent in even a partial return to some measure of self-sufficiency.

Even if we consider only the purely economic returns, it is shortsighted to ignore the resources for economic self-maintenance inherent in the victims of prolonged illness. A large number of them are neither old nor decrepit. They have many years of potential productivity ahead of them, as indicated by studies and by the experience of the Vocational Rehabilitation Administration. Similarly, studies undertaken

[27] "The Geriatric Rehabilitation Service," p. 10.

by the Bureau of Labor Statistics of the United States Department of Labor comparing

Some 11,000 impaired and 18,000 unimpaired workers, subject to the same job incentives and exposed to the same job hazards showed conclusively that the physically impaired worker was not necessarily a handicapped worker. When given reasonable job placement consideration—that is, the individual's abilities balanced against job requirements—the physically impaired workers as a group were fully able to compete successfully with unimpaired workers similarly placed. The two groups had identical frequency rates of nondisabling injuries, and average rates of absenteeism showed only nominal differences. Although the voluntary quit rate was higher for the impaired group, it is questionable whether the difference is large enough to be counted significant.[28]

The availability of facilities to insure the carrying out of an enlightened program of rehabilitation awaits merely the community's recognition of the need and of its obligation to provide for it. Once this is done, it may be possible to help the patient bridge the gap between what he wants for himself and what is possible for him to achieve.

SHELTERED WORKSHOPS

With recognition of the importance of the sheltered workshop as a tool to bring about the gradual return of the disabled to community living came a steady increase in the number of such workshops operated under public and private auspices. These differ as to the diagnostic groups they serve, the facilities they provide, the program they follow, and the standards they maintain. In some, vocational on-the-job training is lacking; many others fail to provide essential comprehensive services or the flexibility necessary to adjust to individual differences. These defects seriously impair the effectiveness of the program and affect negatively the patients' readiness to avail themselves of the services offered.

[28] *The Performance of Physically Impaired Workers in Manufacturing Industries,* pp. 3-4.

The existence of such limitations does not negate the value of sheltered workshops as a means for integrating the disabled person into community living. If this purpose is to be achieved, however, it is essential that a full complement of services be made available. Furthermore, since transportation is a major problem for many of the handicapped, the location of the workshop and ease of access are of primary importance. In fact, some authorities maintain that the sheltered workshop is a vital part of any rehabilitation program without which rehabilitation facilities are incomplete, and have declared that "strategically located rehabilitation centers and sheltered workshops will do much to help solve the problem for many persons with severe physical impairments." [29]

Those of us who are concerned with the provision of total medical care for patients with prolonged illness will agree that a comprehensive rehabilitation program including sheltered workshops where indicated, is essential. The values inherent in such an experience for various levels of disability having been demonstrated, further experimentation and study to determine their maximal usefulness in relation to different diagnostic categories appear to be indicated. Since the effectiveness of sheltered workshops is dependent on the type of program they provide, and the degree to which they are both patient- and community-oriented, it is essential that future planning for these facilities should include provision for setting and maintaining standards.

COMMUNITY ATTITUDES

The recognition of the heavy burden of social and economic pressures imposed by the disabilities of a large number of our citizens has led to definite steps for the establishment of organized rehabilitation facilities as a means of insuring the utilization of their remaining capacites. However, no matter how complete and effective a program may be, no

[29] Elledge, p. 55.

matter what efforts are expended to reeducate and retrain the disabled, in the final analysis their integration into communal life will be determined by the attitude of the community and the extent to which it is ready to offer opportunities for the exercise of newly acquired skills.

As we look about us, we cannot fail to realize that so far the community has made but inadequate provision for the handicapped people in its midst. Our way of living, our housing, our schools, our means of locomotion, our industries, all are geared to serve the average nonhandicapped individual. Usually there is little, if any, attempt to meet the needs of the handicapped.

There is the instance of one woman who had suffered a stroke. Though she was able to navigate slowly with the aid of a cane, she had difficulty in crossing streets. She mentioned that since one of the avenues near her home had been converted to a one-way street in order to expedite traffic, she found it impossible to cross it within the allotted time between light changes. "For people like me," she said, "the island in the middle of the street, where I could wait and be safe, was by far a better arrangement. But then, they do not think of people like me when they make traffic rules."

This lack of concern for the disabled is even more apparent in employment. Despite the experience with disabled workers who were hired during periods of labor shortages and who demonstrated their value in properly selected occupations, despite attempts at education, despite proclamations of "Employ the Handicapped Week," the fear and distrust persist, and the number of employers willing to engage the handicapped is still pitifully small. In the absence of a national emergency employers continue blind to this vast source of potentially useful manpower.

Our greater understanding of the patient's needs and of the significance a job holds for him demands a more thoughtful approach in our attempts at job placement. The stereotyped medical recommendation for hard, medium, or light work, which once seemed sufficient, no longer meets the situation. If work is to enhance the patient's feeling about himself as an adequate, productive member of society, it has to be adjusted not only to the amount of physical exertion of which he is capable, not only to the special skill for which he has been trained, but also to his preferences and the meaning a specific job holds for him. Experience has shown that it is possible not only to find the right job for the right person, but also to adjust the requirements of the job to fit individual needs. By the very nature of the problem he presents, such maximal vocational placement effort for the patient handicapped by prolonged illness is even more important than it admittedly is for the nonhandicapped individual. At the same time, more needs to be done to educate the employer to evaluate the handicapped worker on the basis of his performance rather than his handicap and to eradicate the prejudice against physical deviation from the normal, which is still so greatly in evidence.

A more enlightened approach to the problems of economic productivity for the patient handicapped by the residue of his prolonged illness is important not only for the particular individual concerned, but equally as much for the community as a whole. With the increase in the number of people with prolonged illness who are kept alive by the advances of medical science, large numbers of partially disabled individuals are constantly being added to the community. Unless we learn to utilize constructively this source of manpower inherent in the ever growing older and handicapped population, the burden imposed on the ever smaller proportion of able-bodied young people threatens to affect markedly our national economy and our standard of living. If the experience gained in time of war could be carried over to our peacetime economy, and if the values inherent to the individual and, through him, to the community could be more widely understood, many problems created by the frustration, hopelessness, and feeling of uselessness engendered by enforced idleness could be overcome.

It is indeed encouraging to note that the community is developing, even though slowly, a clearer appreciation of the assets which the handicapped person possesses—assets which can be fruitfully utilized for the benefit of all. What is needed, however, is a more enlightened social philosophy and a more intensive education of the community to the possibility of, and necessity for, utilizing the work capacity of our partially handicapped population, and consequently a recognition and acceptance by the community of the responsibility to provide the necessary facilities to make this possible. Once the need has been recognized, we shall be able to move to a survey of available facilities, an evaluation of their effectiveness, and the creation of such new installations as may be necessary.

A great deal has been said about acute professional personnel shortages as an obstacle to the establishment of extended rehabilitation facilities. There is widespread conviction that without a sufficient number of professionally qualified personnel our newly acquired skills in rehabilitation will not be available to those who need them. No attempt is made to deny the need for more trained personnel. It must be recognized, however, that training personnel is of necessity a long-range project. In the meantime a great deal can be accomplished if we learn to utilize available skills more effectively, to organize the activities of the various members of the rehabilitation team, and to mobilize community resources as well as the innate resources of the patient himself. In this way, we can provide a better preparation for the assimilation of the disabled into the life of the community.

SOCIAL SERVICE AS PART OF TOTAL MEDICAL CARE

The responsibility of the social worker as part of the rehabilitation team was discussed earlier. Her responsibility, however, is not confined to this one area. Since the practice of social medicine is based on the recognition of the importance of social and emotional factors in the treatment of illness, it presupposes the need for coordination of social and medical treatment as integral parts of such care. The application of this philosophy calls for the utilization of the social worker's skills.

Although we have witnessed an expansion of social services in dealing with the problems of illness, the prevailing tendency, nevertheless, is to restrict such services to specific aspects of the healing process and to confine them mainly to those patients who are unable to meet the costs incidental to illness. The concept of total integration of social services as a vital part of all treatment procedures still remains in its infancy.

Prolonged illness, hospitalization, and its sequelae pose numerous and serious problems for all patients. The nature of the problem, however, varies from individual to individual. An understanding of the patient and of the way in which he reacts to the problems that face him is important to all those whose primary obligation is the restoration of the patient to maximal usefulness. One patient may be worried about his financial situation; another may be concerned about his relationship to his family. Still another may be intimidated by the impersonal atmosphere of the hospital, frightened by projected procedures and tests, mystified by his lack of understanding of what is being done and why, bewildered by changes in treatment, frustrated by the slowness of improvement and the threat to his physical well-being, embarrassed by his dependence, resentful of the controls imposed upon him. Whatever the problem, it has its repercussions on the patient's medical condition. Our interest in the total welfare of the patient imposes upon us an obligation to help him to the best of our ability.

In this process of helping, the primary prerequisite is an appreciation of the dignity of the individual and a respect for his rights as a human being, regardless of the stage of his illness or the degree of his impairment. For patients whose illness may leave them with a residual handicap, the need for help extends beyond the period of hospitalization; for it recognizes that the hopes and expectations as well as the anxieties aroused by the preparation for a return to normal living require understanding and skill in handling.

Since we recognize the significance of the close emotional ties which bind members of a family group, and the importance of satisfactory family relationships for the welfare of the patient, the social worker must of necessity be ready to render whatever help may be required by family members. They may need assistance in meeting the problems which the patient's illness creates for them, or help to see the person behind the illness, to have regard for his intrinsic worth, to gear their demands to the limitations imposed by his illness, to utilize imaginatively his remaining potentialities, and to draw him into active participation in family living.

The concept of total medicine extends social service participation beyond direct help to the individual patient and his family into the wider areas of comprehensive medical care through interpretation and research.

In the course of her daily work and by virtue of her close association with the professional team working with the patient, the social worker has an opportunity and an obligation to interpret to its members the social and emotional factors of illness as they affect the patient, his family, and the community. Nor does the need for interpretation end there. The social worker's contacts with the various segments of the community offer an opportunity for sharing her understanding and influencing the thinking of the public about the handicapped individual, his problems, and the importance of utilizing his residual potentialities to the fullest extent.

As a result of her close association with various community groups, the social worker is in a position to make a significant contribution to medical-social research. She can bring to such endeavors a firsthand knowledge of the social problems contributing to, and created by, the illness and can help formulate plans for their amelioration.

Only through such active collaboration in all areas of prevention, treatment, teaching, and research can the goal of social medicine be achieved.

COST OF CARE

No discussion of a program of medical care for prolonged illness can be complete without some consideration of the financial burden it imposes and the ways in which it is being met.

We are all aware that the cost of medical care is steadily increasing. Prolonged illness not only saps the financial resources of the patient and his family, not only interferes with the patient's immediate ability to earn, but, even more frightening, it threatens to curtail his earning capacity for an indefinite period of time—perhaps permanently. The longer the illness, the more permanent the incapacity, the greater is the cost, and the heavier the burden.

In the past the greater share of the cost of hospital care, particularly for patients with prolonged illness, was met either through private philanthropic funds or governmental subsidy. This situation has changed to some degree within recent years.

More and more people are adopting some method of anticipating the financial problem with which illness confronts its victims. Various types of prepaid medical plans have gained public support. Such movements, including group practice units and various voluntary health insurance schemes with ever widening coverage, are constantly expanding, at least among that part of the population which can afford to meet the cost. Employers are assuming more responsibility for participation in plans of health insurance covering their employees. Because of the limitations inherent in these programs, however, they can provide but limited coverage when prolonged illness strikes. The community is thus faced with the necessity of carrying the major part of the burden, either through taxes or through private philanthropy.

This awareness of the need and society's responsibility in meeting it led to the federal Medicare and Medicaid programs enacted in 1965.

Nor is the cost of medical care and hospitalization the whole story. The community must also shoulder a large part of the burden of supporting the temporarily incapacitated or permanently disabled wage earner and his family.

To appreciate the extent of deprivation this can cause, one need only look at the records of public relief agencies and the considerable proportion of chronically ill persons on their rolls. To this must be added a number of others who though not "chronic invalids" are nevertheless forced on public assistance by reason of prolonged illness, or because their residual handicap makes it difficult for them to secure employment. This cost is increasing steadily and constitutes another compelling reason, besides the humanitarian one, to spur our efforts toward better prevention and control of disease and toward a more enlightened policy in the employment of the handicapped.

As we think of the patient with prolonged illness and the problems his illness creates, both when he is suffering from an acute exacerbation of symptoms and during periods of remission, we realize that "the total problem of chronic disease is not a series of separate problems which can be solved one by one, but rather a complex of inter-related problems which require simultaneous actions." [30] Until recently we have done little to mitigate the impact of these problems on the patient, his family, or the community. We have only

[30] "Planning for the Chronically Ill," p. 1265.

begun to think of the facilities necessary for the care of the patient with prolonged illness. We have only begun to take an interest in research, prevention, and early case-finding. We have only begun to appreciate the emotional, familial, and social upheavals such illness creates. We have only begun to see the human being behind the illness and the family behind the patient.

No adequate solution for dealing with the vastness and complexity of these problems has as yet been found. Our knowledge is limited, our facilities woefully inadequate. So much more needs to be known, so much more needs to be done. The significant strides made in medical research give hope of more promising results in the treatment of prolonged illness. The greater awareness of its social implications will of necessity give impetus toward a more inclusive program of care.

A program of care based on our present knowledge has been outlined. Such a program can be of value only if we think of it as a beginning approach to bridge the existing gaps, an approach which must change and grow and evolve as our understanding changes and grows and evolves.

READING REFERENCES

Associated Hospital Service of New York. Annual Report, June, 1962.

Background Facts on the Position of Older Persons. Prepared for the Retirement Income Subcommittee of the Committee on Employment and Retirement of the National Council on the Aging, 1964. Unpublished document.

Bluestone, E. M., M.D. "The Chronic Has a Claim." *Modern Hospital,* LXIII, No. 3 (1944), 67-69.

—— "Long-Term Illness in Modern Society." *Journal of the American Medical Association,* CXXXIII (1947), 1051-53.

—— "Medical Care for Patients with Prolonged Illness." *Annals of the American Academy of Political and Social Science,* CCLXXIII (1951), 144-50.

—— "A Program for Prolonged Illness." *Hospital Management,* LII, No. 5 (1951), 46-49.

—— "Social Medicine Arrives in the Hospital." *Modern Hospital,* LXXV, No. 2 (1950), 59-62, 132.

—— "Some Fundamental Problems in Hospital Administration." *Modern Hospital,* XXIII, No. 6 (1924), 514-18.

—— "These Administrative Axioms." *Modern Hospital,* LXV, No. 2 (1945), 60.

Boas, E. P., M.D. "Clinical Problems." *Proceedings of First Meeting, Commission on Chronic Illness,* May 20, 1949 (Chicago, Commission on the Chronically Ill, 1949), pp. 20-24.

——The Unseen Plague: Chronic Diseases. New York, J. J. Augustin, 1940.

Bourne, W. A., M.D. "An Out-Patients' Club." *Lancet,* CCLVIII (1950) 127-28.

Bracker, Milton. Montefiore Hospital, 1884-1934; a Brief History. New York, privately printed, 1934.

Buchwald, Edith. Physical Rehabilitation for Daily Living. New York, McGraw-Hill, 1952.

Chapman, A. L., M.D. "Implications and Procedures of Multi-phasic Screening." Paper delivered at the 46th Annual Meeting of the National Tuberculosis Association, Washington, D.C., April, 1950. Unpublished document.

—— "Multiple Screening—a New Public Health Technique." Paper delivered at the Annual Meeting of the Tuberculosis and Health Association, Delaware County, Media, Pa., October, 1950. Unpublished document.

Cherkasky, Martin, M.D. "The Montefiore Hospital Home Care Program." *American Journal of Public Health*, XXXIX (1949), 163–66.

"Commission Adopts Further Recommendations on the Care of the Long-Term Patient, The." *Chronic Illness Newsletter*, VI, No. 6 (1955), 1–11.

Covalt, N. K., M.D. "Present and Future Plans for the Rehabilitation of Patients in General Hospitals." *Modern Hospital*, LXXVI, No. 5 (1951), 96–102.

Davis, Milbrew. "Employing the Aged as Foster Grandparents in a Medical Setting," *Social Work Practice, 1966*, pp. 54–60. New York, Columbia University Press, 1966.

Drolet, Godias J., and Donald E. Porter. Why Do Patients in Tuberculosis Hospitals Leave against Medical Advice? Study by the New York Tuberculosis and Health Association (1949). Unpublished document.

Dublin, Louis I., M.D., and Herbert Yahres. "Adding Life to the Added Years." *Collier's*, January 13, 1951, pp. 24–25, 72–73.

Elledge, Caroline H. The Rehabilitation of the Patient. New York, J. B. Lippincott Co., 1948.

Elson, Mildred. "Physical Therapy." *National Council on Rehabilitation Newsletter*, III, No. 7 (1956), 3–7.

Elton, Frederick G. "Rehabilitation, the Place and Relationship of Services." *Rehabilitation Review*, IV, No. 1 (1955), 1–7.

Field, Minna. "Family Sessions: a New Cooperative Step in a Medical Setting." *Journal of Social Casework*, XXX (1949), 417–21.

—— "The Nurse and the Social Worker on the Hospital Team." *American Journal of Nursing*, LV (1955), 695.

Fishbein, Morris, M.D. "Education for Rehabilitation." *Rehabilitation Review*, III, No. 5 (1955), 1–3.

"Geriatric Rehabilitation Service, The." *The Welfarer*, July, 1954, p. 10.

Getting, Vlado A. "A Coordinated State Program for Chronic Illness." *American Journal of Public Health*, XL (1950), 1251–56.

Hinenburg, Morris, M.D. "The Forgotten Patient—How Shall We Plan for Him?" *Modern Hospital*, XL, No. 2 (1933), 73–76.

Hochhauser, Edward. "Objectives of Sheltered Workshops." *Jewish Social Service Quarterly*, XXV (1949), 533–45.

Hospital Council of Greater New York. The Master Plan for Hospitals and Related Facilities for New York City. Annual Report 1958–1959.

Hospital Review and Planning Council of Southern New York. Annual Report 1963–1964.

Jarrett, Mary C. "Preliminary Report on the Chronically Ill Persons Found by a Census in Private Homes for the Aged." Study by the Welfare Council of New York City (1930). Unpublished document.

Kessler, Henry H., M.D. Rehabilitation of the Physically Handicapped. New York, Columbia University Press, 1947.

McNary, Henrietta. "The Scope of Occupational Therapy." Philadelphia, J. B. Lippincott Co., 1947.

New York *Herald Tribune*, March 31, 1950, p. 23.

New York State Department of Social Welfare. Survey of 754 Proprietary Nursing and Boarding Homes for Adults in New York State. 1950. Unpublished document.

New York *Times*, March 21, 1951, p. 35.

Performance of Physically Impaired Workers in Manufacturing Industries, The. A report prepared by the Bureau of Labor Statistics for the Veterans Administration *Bulletin*. No. 923. Washington, D.C., United States Government Printing Office, 1948.

"Planning for the Chronically Ill." *American Journal of Public Health*, XXXVII (1947), 1256–66.

"Position Paper on Education for Nursing," *American Journal of Nursing*, LXV, No. 12 (1965), 106–11.

President's Council on Aging. The Older American. Washington, D.C., Department of Health, Education, and Welfare, 1963.

—— Federal Aid for Nursing Homes, 1963, pp. 1–6.

Ravdin, I. S., M.D. "The Art of Medicine." *New York Medicine,* VII, No. 15 (1951), 22–25.

"Rehabilitation, a Hospital-Community Challenge." *Chronic Illness Newsletter,* II, No. 10 (1951), 1–2.

Richardson, Henry B., M.D. Discussion of Dr. G. Comby Robinson's paper on "Psychosomatic Factors in Convalescence." Convalescent Care (Proceedings of the conference held under the auspices of the Committee on Public Health Relations of the New York Academy of Medicine), pp. 129–49. New York, New York Academy of Medicine, 1940.

—— Patients Have Families. New York, the Commonwealth Fund, 1945.

Rosenfeld, E. D., M.D., *et al.* "Hospital Care Goes Home." *Geriatrics,* VI (1951), 112–16.

Rusk, Howard A., M.D. "Lack of Trained Personnel Felt in Rehabilitation Field." New York *Times,* April 25, 1954, p. 46.

—— "Recovery in Poland." New York *Times,* July 21, 1957, p. 49.

Sayer, Henry D. "Industry and Workmen's Compensation Aspects of Rehabilitation." *Rehabilitation Review,* I, No. 3 (1952), 1–3.

Scheele, Leonard A., M.D. "The Turning Point in Our Care of the Chronically Ill." Proceedings of First Meeting, Commission on Chronic Illness (May 20, 1949), pp. 41–51. Chicago, Commission on Chronic Illness, 1949.

Shapiro, Irving. Health Education in Group Medical Practice with the Health Insurance Plan of Greater New York. Unpublished document.

Shapiro, Sam, *et al.* "Evaluation of Periodic Breast Cancer Screening with Mammography." *Journal of the American Medical Association,* CXCV (1966), 731–38.

Shortley, Michael J. "State Plans for Rehabilitation." *Journal of the American Medical Association,* CXXV (1944), 263–65.

Siltzbach, Louis E. "Relapse and Rehabilitation in the Era of Anti-Tuberculosis Drugs." *Journal of the Mount Sinai Hospital*, XXIII (1956), 635.

Smith, Geddes. Plague on Us. New York, the Commonwealth Fund, 1941.

U.S. Department of Health, Education, and Welfare. Vocational Rehabilitation Administration. Annual Report 1965, p. 276.

U.S. Public Health Service. Characteristics of Patients in Mental Hospitals. National Health Survey. National Center for Health Statistics, Series 12, No. 3. Washington, D.C., 1965.

—— Characteristics of Residents in Institutions for the Aged and Chronically Ill. National Health Survey. National Center for Health Statistics, Series 12, No. 2. Washington, D.C., 1963, p. 10.

—— Chronic Conditions and Activity Limitation. National Health Survey. National Center for Health Statistics, Series 10, No. 17. Washington, D.C., 1965.

—— Hospitalization in the Last Years of Life. National Health Survey. National Center for Health Statistics, Series 22, No. 2. Washington, D.C. 1966.

—— The Magnitude of the Chronic Disease Problem in the United States. National Health Survey. Sickness and Medical Care Series. Preliminary Reports Bulletin No. 6 rev. Washington, D.C., 1939, p. 10.

Weiss, Edward, M.D., and O. Spurgeon English, M.D. Psychosomatic Medicine. 2d ed. Philadelphia, W. B. Saunders Co., 1949.

Weyhmuller, Helen. "Toys at Work." *American Journal of Nursing*, LXV, No. 12 (1965), 68–70.

Whitehouse, Frederick A. "Teamwork: a Democracy of Professions." *Exceptional Children*, XVIII, No. 2 (1951), 45–52.

INDEX

Acute illness: acute stage as phase of prolonged illness, 9; early concentration on acute, 17; *vs.* prolonged, 23, 24, 34, 139, 245-46; effect of advances in medical science, 28

Adjustment after hospitalization, *see* Posthospital adjustment

Adulthood, concept of, 141-42; patient's rights as an adult, 147-55

Age distribution, effect of changes in, 28-31

Aging, *see* Old age

Aging, National Council on, 29

Altro Workshops, New York City, 195, 196, 197; *see also* Sheltered workshops

Alvarez, Walter C., quoted, 80

American Cancer Society, Inc., 27

American Heart Association, Inc., 27

American Hospital Association, 228

American Journal of Gerontology, slogan, 138

American Medical Association, 228

American Nurses' Association, 185; *see also* Nurses

American Public Health Association, 228

American Public Welfare Association, 228

Amputation, traumatic effect of, 72

Antibiotics, effect of development of, 28

Anxieties: at time of hospitalization, 51; of hospitalized children, 61; in cancer patients, 78-79; in tuberculosis, 88; with regard to surgery, 149-51; of family and the home care program, 220

Associated Hospital Service of New York (Blue Cross) *see* Home care program

Bardon-La Follette bill, 169

Blue Cross, *see* Associated Hospital Service of New York, *under* Home care program

Bluestone, E. M., quoted, 9, 21, 35, 56, 60, 146, 261, 264

Blythedale Children's Hospital, Valhalla, N.Y., 69

Boas, E. P., quoted, 234, 244

Bourne, W. A., quoted, 259

Bracker, Milton, quoted, 4

Buchwald, Edith, quoted, 188

Bureau of Labor Statistics, studies of disabled workers, 268

Cancer: in children, 30; as cause of death, 36; fear of diagnosis, 77-82; influence on patient-family relationships, 80, 208-9; early detection of, 236-37; study of early detection of breast cancer, 236-37; detection centers, 236-37; *see also* Multiphasic screening

Cardiovascular diseases, 27, 35; as primary cause of death, 36; largest group in prolonged illnesses, 36

Chapman, A. L., quoted, 238, 239, 240

Charitable organizations: early work in rehabilitation, 168

Chemotherapy, *see* Drug therapy

Cherkasky, Martin, quoted, 131

Children: effect of advances in medical science, 28; prolonged illness among, 30; effect on, of prolonged illness in family, 44-45, 204; evidence of greater concern for their needs, 60-62; hospitalization of, 60-62, 68-69; hospitalization of, and problems of parents, 61-62; Convalescent Hospital, Cincinnati, 68-69; effect of hospitalization on de-

Bei Fragen zur Produktsicherheit wenden Sie sich bitte an:
If you have any questions regarding product safety,
please contact:

Walter de Gruyter GmbH
Genthiner Straße 13
10785 Berlin
productsafety@degruyterbrill.com